Fundamental Clinical Situations

A Practical OSCE Study Guide

PIETER J. JUGOVIC

RICHARD BITAR

LAURA C. McADAM

ELSEVIER
SAUNDERS

Toronto Philadelphia London New York St. Louis Sydney

National Library of Canada Cataloguing in Publication

Jugovic, Pieter J. (Pieter Josef)
    **Fundamental clinical situations : a practical OSCE study guide /
Pieter J. Jugovic, Richard Bitar, Laura C. McAdam. — 4th ed.**

ISBN-13: 978-0-9205-1371-2
ISBN-10: 0-9205-1371-9

    **1. Physical diagnosis—Examinations, questions, etc. 2. Medical
history taking—Examinations, questions, etc. I. Bitar, Richard,
1970- II. McAdam, Laura C. (Laura Catherine), 1972- III. Title.**

RC71.J83 2003   **616.07'5'076**   **C2003-902474-1**

Acquisitions Editor: Ann Millar
Developmental Editor: Francine Geraci
Production Editor: Shefali Mehta
Production Co-ordinators: Kimberly Sullivan, David Ward
Proofreader: Margaret Allen
Cover/Interior Design: Liz Harasymczuk Design
Typesetting and Assembly: Liz Harasymczuk Design
Printing and Binding: Tri-Graphic Printing Limited

Elsevier Canada
905 King St. W., 4th Floor, Toronto, ON, Canada M6K 3G9
Phone: 1-866-896-3331
Fax: 1-866-359-9534

6 7 8 9 10   15 14 13 12 11

Contents

Preface

The first edition of *Fundamental Clinical Situations: A Practical Study Guide* was born from necessity in early spring, 1999, in the Faculty of Medicine at the University of Toronto. Anxiety about our first Objective Standardized Clinical Examination (OSCE) was mounting. Our clinical skills course provided us with the tools we needed to complete histories and physical examinations, and yet we feared that we were not adequately prepared to sit an exam in the format of an OSCE. Could we bring together all the clinical skills we had learned and complete an exam with simulated patient assessments, and do so with rapid efficiency? Like many medical students, we sought a solution from our local bookstore and medical library, but our quest ended in failure, as resources and preparation materials for OSCEs were either not available or not yet written.

It was this void in the medical literature that prompted the creation of a preparatory book, the design of which would allow us to practise our own OSCEs with our peers. This established the primary design of our book as a collection of modules that are scenario-based, each with its own evaluation checklist. The clinical situations were chosen based on their likelihood of appearing on an OSCE, and were created from a variety of references commonly used by medical students.

Two editions followed over the next two years. The breadth of clinical scenarios was increased in each edition in keeping with the broad range of objectives that OSCEs have in medical school and in residency training. Consequently, we developed more clinical scenarios that would test our abilities to complete histories and physical examinations for commonly tested clinical situations. We also designed some challenging psychosocial scenarios, which can throw off medical examinees in high-pressure environments such as OSCEs.

In this latest edition, a total of 68 scenarios have been completed. Many of the checklists and questions following the clinical scenarios have been updated and now reflect current disease-specific, evidence-based guidelines. It is hoped that these improvements will address the preparation for more advanced OSCEs, which are designed to test a student's ability to synthesize information from many sources and then render effective management.

In summary, the book you are about to use contains a collection of clinical modules that are comprehensive in nature and are high-yield for most OSCEs encountered by medical students, internes, and residents during their training. It is based on guidelines where possible. Moreover, it was written by medical students for medical students. And it has been tested at the University of Toronto in three successive editions by medical students who, like you, wanted to ensure their success on OSCEs by finding a resource to help them practise. We hope it serves you well.

Part I

Introduction

AN APPROACH TO THE OSCE

What Is an OSCE?

OSCE is an acronym for Objective Standardized Clinical Examination. It is a test that evaluates a person's clinical performance through simulated patient encounters. The clinical scenarios encountered by candidates are usually common medical complaints or situations. These examinations evaluate:

i.   the ability to elicit a relevant history based on the chief complaint.
ii. the application and successful completion of appropriate, accurate, and safe physical examination manoeuvres, given the chief complaint.
iii. the knowledge and ability to discuss and apply appropriate treatments and potential follow-up with respect to the diagnosis.
iv. the ability to manage difficult patients, including those who present ethical dilemmas.

A Description of Performing an OSCE Station

OSCEs usually begin with the candidate standing outside an examination room. Outside the room, a description—often referred to as a stem—is posted. Read the stem carefully; it presents the clinical case that you will encounter inside, including whether the case is a history, physical, history –physical, or management-based scenario. Do what the stem directs you to do. Should you forget your task, most OSCEs are organized so that the examiners have a copy of the stem in the examination room. Ask to see it if you need to remind yourself of the question. In fact, if you are not addressing the question of your station, your examiner may instruct you to reread the stem. (See "How to Interpret OSCE Stems," below.)

Watch your time carefully, especially if you are to do both an interview and a physical examination. There are usually combinations of signals including bells, whistles, buzzers, etc., that will be explained to you in advance. These signals indicate: starting, passing the mid-point, a wrap-up period, the end of a scenario, and a cue to rotate to the next station. Situations usually vary in length from 5 to 15 minutes, so be efficient with your time. Once you have left a station, leave it behind. Dwelling on a poor performance will only reduce your focus in your next situation.

How to Interpret OSCE Stems

As indicated in the previous section, the stem provides you with enough information to guide your performance at that station. Following is an example of an OSCE stem:

Instructions for Candidate – As an intern doing your internal medicine rotation, you are taking care of Mrs. Pellegrini, a 55-year-old female whom you are treating for congestive heart failure. Today, while you are doing your regular rounds, she tells you that she has felt a lump in her left breast. Perform a directed history and physical examination.

The stem sets the context of the encounter and assumes that the candidate is an intern in internal medicine. This information gives you a clue as to the level of your presumed expertise and the expectations of your performance.

Further, you are provided with the name of a patient, the patient's age, and some past medical information. Write this name down and use it in the exam. Patients appreciate that you know who they are—in an OSCE, and in real life. Addressing a patient appropriately can improve your style and enhance your performance.

Use the patient's age and sex, along with the chief complaint, to write down a differential diagnosis. In this case, you are generating possible causes for a left-breast lump in a female who is most likely postmenopausal.

First, always consider those conditions that are serious or life-threatening—i.e., the "red-flag conditions" that are not to be missed. There are at least one or two red-flag conditions for any given chief complaint, and your questioning and physical examinations should always test for their presence. Examiners watch for questions or physical examination manoeuvres that demonstrate your consideration of the most serious possibilities.

Next, consider the common causes of the chief complaint. Most OSCEs evaluate common clinical conditions. Remember your "horses" and leave out the "zebras" unless you have time. Lastly, consider those conditions about which the patient is concerned. In this case, it is likely that Mrs. Pellegrini is worried about breast cancer. You might use this clue to ask a question such as: "Other female patients I have seen with similar breast lumps have been worried about cancer. What concerns do you have?" This prompt accomplishes a couple of things. First, it may add to your differential diagnosis and focus your questioning and/or the physical examination. Second, it makes the interview patient-centred. A patient-centred approach will go a long way to enhance the evaluation of your interview style.

Finally, the last part of the stem tells you what you are expected to complete. In this case, you will obtain a history and conduct a physical examination. Use this information to budget your time and focus your tasks. If a physical examination is called for, then do not begin with a history. If you forget what was asked of you in the stem, ask to see it again. As mentioned earlier, most OSCEs are set up so that the examiner has a copy of the stem in the room.

The Fundamental Rule Often Forgotten

The fundamental rule that must be remembered by all candidates is that OSCEs also measure the process of the clinical encounter. For example, students often focus on getting all the "checks" in each scenario by blasting through a list of questions or by completing as many examination manoeuvres as possible. However, the way students ask questions and how they complete physical examinations are extremely important also. Do not throw out the "niceties," such as first introducing yourself, explaining to your patients what will take place in the next few minutes, or properly attending to your patients' dignity during physical examinations. You are working against time, but medicine is both a science and an art, and as such, both clinical content and interview style are evaluated in an OSCE. For a guide to the criteria commonly used to evaluate the process or style of OSCEs, please see the section "Global Process Evaluation Criteria."

Also, some of the scenarios that follow have a section reminding you of issues of process. Heed them when practising, and incorporate them into your interviews.

How to Study for OSCEs and Use This Book

A good place to begin preparing for this exam is in the learning objectives of your clinical course. These are usually provided to students at the start of their course work and will provide a framework for the types of clinical situations and physical examination manoeuvres you are expected to master. Other resources include your clinical course instructors and patients on whom you have practised your clinical skills. Feedback from these individuals will highlight your strengths and weaknesses.

However, the best way to prepare for OSCEs is to practise them. Get a partner or small group of friends and simulate the various clinical cases in this book. Take turns playing both examiner and patient. Let your partner, playing the patient, check off each item you complete. Evaluate your performance by adding up all checks in each column. Remember to practise these scenarios in the timeframe for which your exam is set. Most scenarios run between 10 and 20 minutes. Ensure that you also evaluate each other's performance in the Global Evaluation (see "The Fundamental Rule Often Forgotten," above). Answer the questions at the end of the scenario, allotting yourself 5 to 10 minutes. Then, check your answers. Complete other scenarios, and practise often. Soon you will become comfortable with the OSCE format, and your clinical examinations will improve in their focus, accuracy, and rate.

Where to Begin During the OSCE

This section provides a *suggested approach* to directed histories and physical examinations. *It is by no means comprehensive, or even appropriate, for every patient scenario you may experience on an OSCE.* However, it is a good start, especially if you are stumped as to where to begin.

i.   Elicit the identifying data (name, age, marital status, and occupation).
ii.   Elicit the chief complaint.
iii. Generate a differential diagnosis based on the chief complaint.
iv.   Complete the history of the presenting illness by exploring further the chief complaint and associated signs and symptoms, using the differential diagnosis to guide your questions. Remember pertinent negatives to narrow the differential diagnosis. For example, ask the following questions:

L DOCC SPARC CIP

- Location — Where is the chief complaint experienced?
- Duration — How long does the chief complaint last?
- Onset — When did the chief complaint start?
- Course — What are the changes in the chief complaint over time?
- Character — Describe the quantity and quality of the chief complaint.
- Severity — Grade the chief complaint on a scale from 0 (no pain) to 10 (worst pain the patient can imagine) both for its time of onset and for the present.
- Palliating/Provoking — What makes the chief complaint better and worse?
- Associated S&S — What are the signs and symptoms presenting as a complex with the chief complaint?
- Risk Factors — What are the factors known to enhance chances of having the chief complaint?
- Constitutional Signs — Fever, chills, night sweats, changes in sleep, energy level, weight, and appetite.
- Causation — What does the patient think the cause is?
- Impact on the Patient — How has the illness affected the patient?
- Patient's Action — What has the patient done for the complaint(s)? Medications?

v. Inquire about the patient's past medical history, including:

SHIAMS

- Surgeries — Type, when, outcome(s).
- Hospitalizations — Condition, when hospitalized, outcome(s).
- Illnesses — In adults, always ask about HTN, DM, Hx of cancer, as well as duration and treatments.
- Allergies — Drugs, description of reaction(s), MedAlert?, EpiPen?
- Medications — Types and dosing.
- Sins — Smoking/alcohol/drug use.

vi. If required, midway through the session begin the necessary physical examinations. Describe what you are doing and the clinical findings you see (or might see), given the chief complaint. You might do this by explaining these findings (or potential findings) to your patients while you are examining them. This involves them in the encounter and demonstrates your attentiveness. Ultimately, this approach will enhance your process evaluation.

vii. Remember to help the patient re-robe, if necessary, then summarize and conclude the interview in the wrap-up period. This step is important even if it means forgoing additional lines of questioning or examinations, as it contributes to style. It is always very poor form to leave the room while in mid-question or mid-examination because your time is up. Obviously, a summary is much more appealing and may serve to remind the marker about the points covered that may not have been checked off.

Post-Encounter Probes (PEPs)

Some OSCEs have questions in written format. Some are asked by an examiner. You may be asked any of the following questions: "What is the diagnosis?," "What is your differential diagnoses?," "What are some risk factors for this disease?," "What diagnostic tests should be ordered?," or "What are the next steps in treatment?" In more advanced OSCEs, data from investigations are used. For example, it is not uncommon to be asked to interpret test results such as chest x-rays, CTs or MRIs of the head, EKGs, pulmonary function tests, and blood results. If you have prepared well for your OSCE, PEPs are a straightforward means of boosting your evaluation.

Important Hints

- Most OSCEs will not allow you to bring any written material into the exam. However, blank paper is usually provided just before you start so that you can jot down notes during each interview. After you have read the stem of the encounter you are about to start, use this paper to write down L DOCC SPARC CIP and SHIAMS to prompt your memory if you get stuck. It is also helpful to write down a differential diagnosis for each scenario, so that you focus your questions and/or physical examinations to rule these possibilities in or out.
- As a means of identifying the exam candidates, OSCEs use identification stickers at each station. Before you start the exam, you might consider folding the corner up on all your stickers, making it easier and faster to give them to the examiner before the interview starts.
- There are some situations that, because of logistics, are very unlikely to appear on OSCEs. Examples include pelvic and rectal examinations and examinations involving babies or small children. However, you may have to interview a mother concerning her baby, and use growth charts or make observations from pictures of children.
- Breast examinations often appear on OSCEs. Know a differential for breast lumps and risk factors for breast cancer. Examinations of the back, shoulder, hip, and knee are also very popular.
- Scan the room when you first enter it. There may be equipment or props that you need to use in your physical examinations. Examples include otoscopes, ophthalmoscopes, BP cuffs, reflex hammers, latex gloves, tongue depressors, cotton, glasses of water, growth charts, pictures of patients, etc. These items are clues to the tasks that need to be completed. For example, a glass of water is almost always used in a thyroid examination, a piece of cotton in a sensory examination, and so on. Usually, examiners do not bring your attention to these items, so you might miss out if you do not take note of them yourself.
- Use universal precautions. If your examination involves possible contact with blood, use gloves, which may be provided, or at least indicate to the examiner that you would use gloves before you start.

An examination of the hand with a simulated palm laceration is an example of a case where universal precautions must be used on an OSCE.

- Any equipment you are asked to bring, such as stethoscopes, reflex hammers, pen lights, ophthalmoscopes, and otoscopes, will be used in some way on the exam. Know how to use the items you are required to have. Make sure they are in working order the night before the OSCE, including recharging the batteries.
- Ask your upperclassmen and women what types of cases they encountered on past OSCEs and what challenges they faced. This suggestion is tempered with a warning. Students are often tempted to find out about OSCEs from their classmates who might have just taken the exam. *This can be a trap!* While anxious students see it as a means of survival, your administration could view this as academic dishonesty in both parties involved. In addition, your examiners will alter the diagnosis in various clinical situations in different sessions of the exam. For example, right-lower-quadrant abdominal pain in a young female on day 1 of the OSCE could be appendicitis, but on day 2 it could easily be changed to ectopic pregnancy. Base your approach and diagnosis on what you determine clinically from the history and the physical examination, and also on any results of investigations that are provided. Avoid making a diagnosis based on answers from previous exam sessions.
- Concentrate on common manoeuvres in physical examinations. For example, noting the presence of Frank's sign in a person with crushing chest pain will not be as high-yielding as noting the JVP or doing a precordial examination. Medical trivia are great for impressing your medical preceptors, but are probably low-yield on OSCEs.
- When doing physical examinations, you must describe everything you are doing and seeing or expect to see. Occasionally, the examiner will not be able to appreciate the signs or symptoms you elicit. Thus, you must clarify your progress by describing each manoeuvre and its corresponding finding. You might explain these findings to the patient you are examining as a means of making the encounter patient-centred, rather than phrasing them in the third person. This approach will enhance your process mark. Also, be honest in reporting your results. If you do not appreciate a finding but know you should, given the case, then indicate this. No one will ever fault you for your honesty. By saying aloud what you would expect to find, given the chief complaint, you will have demonstrated sound knowledge.
- If you get stumped or freeze up—relax. Ask the patient to give you a moment to collect your thoughts. Restart by summarizing the data you have so far. This strategy may jog your memory and prompt new questions or examinations. It also gives the appearance to your examiner that you are organized.
- If you finish an OSCE station early, know that the examiner and patient will not engage you in conversation. This allows you to

re-enter the clinical situation at a later time with more questions or examination manoeuvres as needed. If you cannot think of more to ask or do, then just sit quietly and wait out your time. You are not allowed to leave the room and rotate to the next station, as this will disrupt the flow of the exam for the rest of the candidates.

- Remember to go to the washroom just before the exam. Nothing is worse than having to urinate when you arrive at your second station. Before the start of the exam, eat and drink well, as OSCEs can be long and are demanding physically and intellectually. Also, remember to get a good night's rest before the exam.
- Dress appropriately and comfortably. This usually means clothes that you would wear when seeing patients in clinic or on the wards, and includes a lab coat.
- The worst part of the OSCE is the wait before it starts. Once you get over the initial anxiety, the exam will flow and be over before you know it.

Global Process Evaluation Criteria

Opening
☐ i.   Greeted patient and introduced self.
☐ ii. Ascertained patient's name and elicited chief complaint.

Interpersonal Skills
☐ i.   Used proper eye contact and body posture.
☐ ii. Was aware of and responded to the patient's nonverbal cues and emotional content.
☐ iii. Use of silence and interruptions was appropriate.
☐ iv. Used reflection, checked accuracy of understanding.

Information Gathering
☐ i.   Asked one question at a time and avoided jargon.
☐ ii.   Used both open-ended and directed questions.
☐ iii. Questions asked were appropriate for scenario.
☐ iv. Questions asked were logical and ordered.
☐ v.   Controlled pace of interview.
☐ vi. Clarified and summarized appropriately.
☐ vii. Ensured that patient understood questions asked.
☐ viii. Ensured that patient's concerns were addressed and closed interview.
☐ ix. Showed evidence of hypothesis testing to narrow a diagnosis.

Physical Examination
☐ i.   Ensured patient was suitably dressed for the exam.
☐ ii.   Patient's privacy was considered, used draping, curtains, etc.
☐ iii. Used proper lighting.
☐ iv. Positioned self to perform physical manoeuvres with ease.
☐ v.   Positioned patient to observe symmetry, perform manoeuvres, etc.
☐ vi. Was considerate and gentle when examining the patient.
☐ vii. Restored patient's clothing, position, etc., after examination.

The global scoring criteria are self-explanatory. They should be employed for each scenario that is practised. Each of the evaluations that follow will examine the content of a specific clinical situation, but the global scoring criteria evaluate the style of both the interview and the physical examination. The content and style are equally important, and thus each constitutes one-half of an interviewer's score. Pay particular attention to sections (iii) and (ix) in the "Information Gathering" section.

Part II

Scenarios for Directed Histories

Evaluation: History for Amenorrhea

INSTRUCTIONS FOR CANDIDATE

You are a family physician in a busy practice. One of your patients, Sarah Ali, a 24-year-old female, has booked a morning appointment with you because over the past few months she has not had her menstrual cycle. Perform a directed history.

EVALUATION CRITERIA

I. History

i. Menses
- ❏ Age at Onset of Menses
- ❏ Length of Period
- ❏ Regularity of Period
- ❏ Last Menstrual Period
- ❏ Menstrual Cramping

ii. Obstetric and Gynecologic
- ❏ Current Sexual Activity
- ❏ Safe Practices and Contraception (frequency of use, types)
- ❏ Symptoms of Pregnancy (nausea, vomiting, breast pain, urinary frequency, fatigue)
- ❏ Intrauterine Adhesions (previous dilation and curettage, pelvic infection)

iii. Endocrine (Screens for Symptoms of)
- ❏ Hypothyroidism (cool and dry skin, cold intolerance, constipation, fatigue, weakness)
- ❏ Hyperthyroidism (warm and soft skin, heat intolerance, diarrhea, tremor)
- ❏ Hypoestrogenism (hot flashes, night sweats)
- ❏ Prolactinoma (galactorrhea, visual changes, headache)
- ❏ Hyperandrogenism (acne, hirsutism, temporal balding, deepening of voice)
- ❏ Hyperglucocorticoidism (centripetal obesity, striae, hirsutism, supraclavicular fat pad)

iv. Past Medical History
- ❏ Excessive Dieting/Eating Disorder
- ❏ Excessive Exercise
- ❏ Current Illnesses
- ❏ Genetic Abnormalities (Turner's syndrome, testosterone insensitivity)

- ❏ Psychological Stressors
- ❏ Current Medications (birth control pill, marijuana, phenothiazine, antidepressants, chemotherapy, radiation)

POST-ENCOUNTER PROBE

Q1. What is the difference between primary and secondary amenorrhea?

Primary amenorrhea occurs in females who have not had an onset of menses by age 15. Secondary amenorrhea is the cessation of menses for more than 3 consecutive cycles or for more than 6 months in women who previously had normal menstruation.

Q2. Identify 15 causes of amenorrhea.

Anatomic—pregnancy, intrauterine adhesions, gonadal dysgenesis, imperforate hymen, vaginal septum

Ovarian Failure—menopause, surgery, radiation, chemotherapy, chromosomal abnormalities (Turner's syndrome, androgen insensitivity), resistant ovary syndrome

Endocrine—hypo/hyperthyroidism, Cushing's disease, hyperandrogenism (polycystic ovarian disease, ovarian or adrenal tumour, testosterone injections), hyperprolactinoma, hypothalamic or pituitary tumours

Miscellaneous—stress, eating disorder, post OCP, illness, excessive exercise, low percentage of body fat

Q3. What investigations could you order to help diagnose the cause of this patient's amenorrhea? Justify each test.

β-HCG—to determine if there are products of conception present

TSH, T3—to determine if there is hypo- or hyperthyroidism present

Prolactin—to determine if pituitary tumour is present

Progesterone Challenge—to determine estrogen status

FSH and LH—to determine whether there is ovarian failure or hypothalamic dysfunction

U/S—to rule out polyovarian syndrome, structural obstruction

Karyotype—to determine genetic abnormality, e.g., Turner's syndrome, androgen insensitivity syndrome

Evaluation: History for Anemia

INSTRUCTIONS FOR CANDIDATE

You are a physician at a walk-in clinic. Your nurse informs you that your next patient, Samantha Lui, 32, is here because she has had increasing fatigue and heart palpitations and thinks that she looks pale. Perform a directed history.

EVALUATION CRITERIA

I. **History**

   i. **Fatigue**
- ❏ Duration
- ❏ Onset
- ❏ Course
- ❏ Frequency
- ❏ Limitations in Activities

   ii. **Associated Symptoms**
- ❏ Malaise
- ❏ Weakness
- ❏ Dyspnea
- ❏ Chest Pain
- ❏ Palpitations
- ❏ Headache
- ❏ Tinnitus
- ❏ Presyncope/Syncope

   iii. **Potential Sites of Blood Loss**
- ❏ Past Anemias
- ❏ Menstrual Bleeds (changes in frequency, amount, duration of menses)
- ❏ Lower Resp. Tract Bleeds (hemoptysis)
- ❏ Upper Resp. Tract Bleeds (epistaxis)
- ❏ Lower GI Bleeds (melena, hematochezia)
- ❏ Upper GI Bleeds (hematemesis)
- ❏ Urinary/Renal Bleeds (hematuria)
- ❏ Past Blood Donations (frequency, last donation, amount donated)

   iv. **Other Etiologies of Anemia**
      Dietary History:
- ❏ Iron Deficiency
- ❏ Folic Acid/B_{12} Deficiency

      Past Medical History:
- ❏ Chronic Inflammatory Disorders
- ❏ Liver or Renal Disease

- ☐ Endocrine Disorders (hypo/hyperthyroid, Addison's disease)
- ☐ Malignancies (myeloma, leukemia)
- ☐ Alcohol Use (quantity, duration)
- ☐ Lead Exposure
- ☐ Medications (NSAIDs, chemotherapeutic agents)

Family Medical History:
- ☐ Genetic Background (Mediterranean/African/Asian)
- ☐ Hereditary Anemia (sideroblastosis, spherocytosis, elliptocytosis, stomatocytosis)

POST-ENCOUNTER PROBES

Q1. Provide an approach to the differential diagnosis of anemia.

Microcytic Anemia (MCV<80)
Iron deficiency, thalassemia, lead poisoning, sideroblastic disease, chronic illness

Normocytic Anemia (MCV = 80 – 100)
i.   Low Reticulocytes
Myelodysplasia, myelofibrosis, aplasia, marrow infiltration (leukemia, metastasis, infection), liver disease, uremia, hypo- or hyperthyroidism, Addison's disease, chronic illness
ii. High Reticulocytes
- Bleeding
- Hemolysis — spherocytosis, elliptocytosis, stomatocytosis, G6PD deficiency, PK deficiency, sickle-cell disease, S-thalassemia, TTP, ITP, DIC, HUS, heart valve disease, burns, transfusion reaction, HIV infection, systemic lupus, lymphoma

Macrocytic Anemia (MCV >100)
- B_{12} or folate deficiency, drug reaction, myelodysplasia, bone marrow infiltration or suppression, liver disease, asplenia, alcoholism, hypothyroidism, erythropoietin treatment, selenium deficiency, Trisomy 21 (Down syndrome)

Q2. For severe or symptomatic anemia, it is often necessary to transfuse packed red blood cells. What are the potential complications of transfusions?

Hemolytic Reactions
i.   Major hemolytic transfusion reaction
ii. Minor hemolytic transfusion reaction
iii. Delayed hemolytic transfusion reaction

Nonhemolytic Reactions
i.   Acute allergic reactions
ii. Acute febrile reactions

iii.   Graft-versus-host reactions

iv.   Infections — HIV, Human T-cell Leukemia/Lymphoma Virus-1, cytomegalovirus, hepatitis B/C

v.   Iron overload

Q3. What initial investigations would you order in an anemic patient?

CBC, serum ferritin, reticulocyte count, blood film

Evaluation: History for Benign Prostatic Hyperplasia (BPH)

INSTRUCTIONS FOR CANDIDATE

Jerome Blackhart is a 61-year-old man who made an appointment with his family doctor because he is very tired, as he has been waking several times at night to go to the bathroom. You are doing a locum for his family doctor. Perform a directed history.

EVALUATION CRITERIA

I. **History**

   i. **BPH**

      Obstructive

- ❑ Hesitancy
- ❑ Diminished Force of Stream
- ❑ Intermittence
- ❑ Postvoid Dribbling
- ❑ Suprapubic Pain or Fullness

      Irritative

- ❑ Urgency
- ❑ Dysuria
- ❑ Frequency
- ❑ Nocturia

   ii. **Associated Symptoms**

- ❑ Incontinence
- ❑ Urinary Infections
- ❑ Erectile Dysfunction
- ❑ Systemic (fever, chills, etc.)

POST-ENCOUNTER PROBES

Q1. a. How is the prostate gland examined?

Digital rectal examination (DRE)

b. What are the contraindications for this exam?

Neutropenia; a patient who lacks an anus, an examiner who lacks digits. In other words, always do a DRE unless the patient is neutropenic.

c. What is the protein screened for in lab tests?

PSA (prostate-specific antigen)

Q2. a. Prostatic hyperplasia occurs in what area of the prostate in a large majority of patients?

Periurethral area

b. Which area of the prostate is affected for the majority of malignancies of the prostate?

Peripheral zone, which is amenable to the DRE

Q3. A nodule found on the prostate during a DRE is not always malignant. Provide a differential diagnosis of prostatic nodule.

- Prostatic Cancer
- Benign Prostatic Hyperplasia
- Prostatic Calculus
- Chronic Prostatitis
- Tuberculous Prostatitis

Evaluation: History for Diabetes

INSTRUCTIONS FOR CANDIDATE

You are a medical student in a multidisciplinary medical clinic. Your preceptor has asked you to see Geraldine Jeffery, a 60-year-old woman with Type II diabetes. Perform a directed history.

EVALUATION CRITERIA

I.   History — Acute Complications
  i.   Hyperglycemia
- ❏ Polyphagia
- ❏ Weight Changes
- ❏ Polydipsia (+/– nocturia)
- ❏ Polyuria
- ❏ Blurry Vision
- ❏ Yeast Infections

  ii. Hypoglycemia
- ❏ Adrenergic S&S
- ❏ Hunger
- ❏ Palpitations
- ❏ Sweating
- ❏ Anxiety
- ❏ Tremors
- ❏ Seizures

II. History — Chronic Complications
  i.   Macrovascular Changes
- ❏ Stroke
- ❏ Coronary Artery Disease
- ❏ Peripheral Vascular Disease

  ii. Microvascular Changes
- ❏ Retinopathy (loss of vision)
- ❏ Cataracts
- ❏ Sensory: Paresthesia (glove-and-stocking distribution)
- ❏ Motor: Motor Deficits
- ❏ Impotence
- ❏ Neuropathy (Autonomic)
- ❏   Orthostatic Hypotension

- ❏   Gastroparesis
- ❏   Diarrhea
- ❏   Voiding Difficulties
- ❏   Nephropathy
- ❏   Hypertension

III.   Risk Factors
- ❏   Family Hx of DMII
- ❏   Gestational Diabetes
- ❏   Dyslipidemia
- ❏   Hypertension
- ❏   Central Obesity

IV.   Management and Control
i.   Diet
- ❏   Caloric Intake
- ❏   Am't and Types of Fats, Protein, Fibre, and Sugar

ii.   Lifestyle
- ❏   Weight
- ❏   Smoking
- ❏   Alcohol or Substance Use
- ❏   Exercise (type and amount)

iii.   Drug Treatments
- ❏   Medications
- ❏   Hypoglycemic Agents (type, frequency, side effects)
- ❏   Insulin (type, amount, dosing schedule, side effects)
- ❏   Monitoring (type [blood/urine], frequency, HbA_{1c})
- ❏   Adherence to Recommendations

POST-ENCOUNTER PROBES

Q1. How is diabetes mellitus diagnosed?

i.   Symptoms of diabetes mellitus (polyuria, polydipsia, fatigue, weight loss) + random blood glucose >11.1 mmol/L

OR

ii.   Fasting blood glucose >7.0 mmol/L

OR

iii.   Fasting blood glucose in 2-h sample of oral glucose tolerance test >11.1

(i), (ii), (iii), or some combination of these on two different days. Re-testing is not necessary if there was hyperglycemia plus acute metabolic decompensation.

Q2. Describe the chronic neurological pathologies that occur in many diabetic patients.

Autonomic Neuropathy—orthostatic hypotension, gastroparesis (nausea, vomiting, postprandial bloating and early satiety), neurogenic bladder (retention and overflow incontinence), and impotence

Sensory Neuropathy—vibration sense (first lost), proprioception and light touch in glove-and-stocking distribution, Charcot's joints, foot ulcerations

Radiculopathy—shooting or burning pain, often radiating down lower extremities

Mononeuropathy—cranial nerve palsies; often CNIII (but pupils spared), CNIV, CNVI

Amyotrophy—atrophy of the pelvic girdle and large leg muscles that can spontaneously remit. Often affects older males

Mononeuritis Multiplex—peripheral nerve palsies that can cause sensory or motor neuropathies such as foot drop

Q3. a. What are the clinical features of diabetic ketoacidosis (DKA)?

Usually, a young patient with Type I DM experiencing polyuria, polydipsia, loss of consciousness, anorexia, nausea, vomiting, fatigue, abdominal pain, or Kussmaul's breathing

b. What are the clinical precipitants of DKA?

DKA may be precipitated by infection, noncompliance with taking proper insulin dose, initial presentation of Type I diabetes, or idiopathic causes.

Q4. Take a systems-based approach and describe physical manoeuvres that one should observe in a diabetic patient.

General—height, weight, waist circumference, BMI, orthostatic blood pressure, pulse

Head and Neck—pupil reactions, fundi, lens opacity, extraocular movements, oral hygiene, thyroid

Cardiovascular—signs of congestive heart failure, pulses, bruits

Abdomen—organomegaly

Musculoskeletal—foot inspection for skin changes and ulcers; joint mobility and hand inspection for arthropathy

Central Nervous System—changes in vibration, proprioception, light touch and reflexes, autonomic neuropathy

Skin—cutaneous infections, signs of dyslipidemias

Q5. Describe the tests one should do and their timing in routine follow-up visits for diabetes mellitus.

- Directed diabetic histories, blood pressure, and foot examination every 2–4 months
- Glycated hemoglobulin every 2–4 months, fasting glucose levels as needed
- Fasting lipid profile every 12 months
- Dipstick of urine for gross proteinuria every 6–12 months. If positive, creatinine clearance and microalbuminuria every 6–12 months. If negative, albumin:creatinine ratio every 12 months. Resting EKG every 12 months if >35 years old

Q6. a. What are the potential therapies one can use to treat Type II diabetics?

Nonpharmacologic—diet changes, exercise, weight loss, reduction of alcohol use. If unsuccessful within 2–4 months, advance to:

Monotherapy with Oral Agents—alpha-glucosidase inhibitor, biguanides, sulfonylurea. If unsuccessful within 2–4 months, advance to:

Combination Oral Therapy—alpha-glucosidase inhibitor, biguanides, and sulfonylureas. Maximize to upper limits of the drug over 2–4 months before moving to next class of medications. New insulin secretagogues, such as repaglinide or gliclazide, and peripheral-tissue insulin potentiators, such as the thiazolidinediones, are new alternatives in oral hypoglycemics. They might be used in combination therapies. If unsuccessful within 2–4 months, advance to bedtime insulin or daily insulin regimes.

Bedtime Insulin—intermediate-acting insulin (NPH, lente) with combination of oral agents. If unsuccessful within 2–4 months, advance to:

Insulin Injections—2–4 injections each day. Occasionally, oral agents including metformin, rosiglitazone, or acarbose are used with insulin.

b. When should biguanides such as metformin not be used?

Contraindications include renal or hepatic failure, hypersensitivity to the drug, metabolic acidosis, CHF, acute MI, and concomitant use of iodinated contrast.

Q7. Give four helpful pieces of advice for a diabetic patient regarding exercise.

i. Use proper footwear; inspect your feet daily and after exercise. Use protective footwear as needed.
ii. Avoid exercise over periods of unstable metabolic control.
iii. Take blood sugar readings before start of exercise and consume simple, rapidly absorbed carbohydrates if blood sugar <5.
iv. Avoid exercise in extreme hot or cold conditions.
v. Administer insulin into a site away from those muscle groups being exercised.

Q8. *Give advice to a diabetic patient about managing diabetic therapies and sick days.*

i.   Always take your insulin or hypoglycemic agent, though the dosage may need adjusting by your doctor.
ii. Try to follow your meal plan if you can eat.
iii. Drink plenty of water to prevent dehydration.
iv. Test your blood sugar every 2–4 hours. If you sense it is low, then test more frequently.
v.   Test your urine or blood for ketones.
vi. Seek medical attention from a doctor if:
   a. you have been vomiting or having diarrhea for >4 h.
   b. you are unable to eat or drink.
   c. your blood sugar is >17 mmol/L for more than 12 h.
   d. you have moderate to large amounts of ketones in your urine or >1.5 mmol/L blood ketones.
   e. you show signs of dehydration, including a dry mouth, cracked lips, dry skin, or sunken eyes.
   f. your chest hurts, your breath smells fruity, you are having trouble breathing, or you cannot think clearly.
   g. you are not certain what to do to take care of yourself or have questions or worries about your symptoms or illness.

Evaluation: History for Diarrhea

INSTRUCTIONS FOR CANDIDATE

You are an emergency physician in a rural emergency room. Your next patient has presented with a 4-day history of diarrhea. Her name is Margaret Sharp, and she is 29 years old. Perform a directed history.

EVALUATION CRITERIA

I. History

  i. Diarrhea
- ❏ Timing (duration, onset, and course)
- ❏ Quantity
- ❏ Quality
- ❏ Frequency
- ❏ Aggravating/Alleviating Factors

  ii. Associated Symptoms
- ❏ Fever
- ❏ Weight Loss
- ❏ Change in Appetite and Diet
- ❏ Vomiting
- ❏ GI/Nausea
- ❏ Urination
- ❏ Tenesmus
- ❏ Melena
- ❏ Hematochezia

  iii. Risk Factors
- ❏ Travel History
- ❏ Outbreak (friends/family)
- ❏ Seafood (food poisoning)
- ❏ Extra GI (eye, skin, and joint)
- ❏ Family Hx (IBD, bowel cancer)
- ❏ Diet Changes
- ❏ Laxative Use
- ❏ Steatorrhea
- ❏ Celiac Disease
- ❏ Lactose Intolerance
- ❏ Immunosuppressed
- ❏ Medications and Allergies
- ❏ Anal Intercourse

POST-ENCOUNTER PROBES

Q1. a. Name one viral,

Rotavirus, Norwalk virus, adenovirus, togavirus

b. one bacterial, and

E. coli (EHEC, EPEC, ETEC), *Shigella*, *Campylobacter*, *Yersinia*, *Salmonella*, Clostridia

c. one parasitic pathogen that can cause diarrhea.

E. histolytica, Giardia

Q2. Explain how Clostridium difficile *can cause pseudomembranous colitis in a patient with a history of antibiotic use.*

Antibiotics deplete regular gut flora, which normally outnumber *C. difficile*. *C. difficile* can resist antibiotics as a spore and then will outgrow normal flora when antibiotics are discontinued. Toxins A and B produced by the greater numbers of *C. difficile* cause diarrhea.

Q3. If you suspected the patient was dehydrated from the diarrhea, give four signs and symptoms that would confirm your suspicion.

Complaints of dry mucous membranes (eyes, mouth, etc.), thirst, sunken eyes, tachypnea, tachycardia, decreased JVP, decreased skin turgor, decreased urination, decreased weight, irritability/lethargy, low blood pressure

Q4. a. Name the psychiatric eating disorder associated with the misuse of laxatives.

Bulimia nervosa

b. If you suspected this disorder, what three clinical features could confirm your suspicions?

Any three of the following: hypothermia, bradycardia, arrhythmias, dry skin, languor, hair loss, scars or calluses on the dorsum of hand, loss of dental enamel, large parotid glands, pedal edema

Q5. During the patient history, how could one identify diarrhea caused by a problem in the small bowel?

A problem in the small bowel will cause a problem with absorption; therefore, inquire as to history of weight loss, weakness, and steatorrhea. May also see fat-soluble vitamin deficiencies such as night blindness, dry skin, bone disease (rickets), anemia, neurological disorders, and bleeding disorders.

Q6. Provide a means of classifying acute and chronic diarrhea.

Acute (<2 wks):
Inflammatory — bacterial, parasitic, IBD (S&S: blood, pain, fever)
Noninflammatory — viral, food poisoning, fecal impaction

Chronic (>2 wks):
Inflammatory — bacterial, parasitic, IBD, ischemic colitis
Osmotic — lactose intolerance, pancreatic insufficiency, celiac sprue
Secretory — bacteria, toxins, laxatives
Hypersecretion — functional (IBS, laxatives), hyperthyroid

Evaluation: History for the Elderly

INSTRUCTIONS FOR CANDIDATE

As a family physician, you have been concerned about Mary MacDonald, a 92-year-old woman, who has come into your office two days late for her scheduled appointment. You notice she is wearing food-stained clothes. Assess her functional capacity and ability to cope independently by performing a directed history.

EVALUATION CRITERIA

I. **History**

  i. **Functional Assessment**
    ADLs:
- ❏ Transfers
- ❏ Dressing
- ❏ Bathing
- ❏ Toileting
- ❏ Food Preparation
- ❏ Stairs
- ❏ Walking

    IADLs:
- ❏ Cooking
- ❏ Cleaning
- ❏ Laundry
- ❏ Shopping
- ❏ Paying Bills
- ❏ Driving

  ii. **Geriatric Giants**
- ❏ Falls
- ❏ Fractures
- ❏ Confusion
- ❏ Medications
- ❏ Incontinence (bowel and bladder)

  iii. **Sensorium**
- ❏ Sight
- ❏ Hearing
- ❏ Balance

  iv. **Social Factors**
- ❏ Marital Status
- ❏ Living Arrangements

- ❏ Family Support
- ❏ Community/Medical Resources Used
- ❏ Advance Directives/Living Will

v. Mood
- ❏ Assesses Mood (determines changes, severity of changes)
- ❏ Assesses Aggravating/Alleviating Factors
- ❏ Assesses Suicidality
- ❏ Assesses Homicidality

vi. Anxiety Symptoms
- ❏ Anxiety/Panic Attacks Experienced
- ❏ Phobias (What are patient's fears?)
- ❏ Obsessions (Persistent thoughts in mind?)
- ❏ Compulsions (Persistent actions he/she must do?)

vii. Perception
- ❏ Hallucinations (Do you ever hear/see things others don't?)
- ❏ Delusions (Do you feel the TV/radio is speaking to you?)
- ❏ Derealizations (Do you ever feel the world is not real?)
- ❏ Depersonalization (Do you ever feel you're someone else?)

viii. Folstein Mini-Mental Status Exam
- ❏ Orientation (place, time: 5 pt for each)
- ❏ Registration (name 3 objects: 1 pt for each)
- ❏ Attention/Concentration (serial 7's, world, months: 5 pt total)
- ❏ Recall (recall 3 objects: 1 pt for each)
- ❏ Language
- ❏ (identify 2 objects pointed to: 2 pt total)
- ❏ (ask no ifs, ands, or buts: 1 pt total)
- ❏ (perform 3-stage command: 3 pt total)
- ❏ (read and obey written command: 1 pt total)
- ❏ (write a sentence: 1 pt total)
- ❏ (draw intersecting pentagons: 1 pt total)

II. Process Evaluation*

i. Interpersonal Skills
- ❏ Was aware of patient's nonverbal cues and emotional content
- ❏ Used reflection, checked accuracy of understanding

ii. Information Gathering
- ❏ Asked one question at a time and avoided jargon
- ❏ Used both open-ended and directed questions
- ❏ Clarified and summarized appropriately
- ❏ Ensured that patient understood questions asked
- ❏ Ensured that patient's concerns were addressed and closed interview

*See Global Process Evaluation Criteria (page 10) for a complete evaluation of the interview process.

POST-ENCOUNTER PROBES

Q1. Falls are common causes of accidents and morbidity in seniors. Give three physiologic and three pathologic reasons for this.

Physiologic	Pathologic
• Decreased visual acuity	• Cardiac: MI, orthostatic hypotension
• Decreased night vision	• Neurological: stroke, TIA, dementia, Parkinson's disease
• Diminished sensory awareness, touch	• Metabolic: hypoglycemia, anemia, dehydration
• Increased body sway, impaired righting mechanisms	• MSK: arthritis, muscle weakness
	• Drug-induced: diuretics, antihypertensives

Q2. Why might elderly females be at higher risk for fractures?
Osteoporosis often elevates the risk of fractures in the elderly, especially females.

Q3. Your 92-year-old patient had suffered a fall from an undetermined cause while living alone at home. Describe two possible complications.
- Soft-tissue injuries resulting in decreased function
- Fractures involving the hip or wrist (Colles' fracture)
- Subdural hematoma
- Long-term complications including reduction in ADLs and IADLs for physical reasons, or psychological ones, should the senior fear falling again

Q4. Describe three reasons why a senior may have urinary incontinence.
DRIP
Delirium/Diabetes mellitus (hyperglycemia)
Restricted mobility/Retention
Infections (UTI)/Impaction of Stool
Psychological/Pills (long-acting sedatives, diuretics, anticholinergic agents)

Q5. If a fall had occurred, what information would you want to elicit from the patient and/or from bystanders who may have witnessed the fall?
- Activity at the time of the fall
- Symptoms before and after the fall, such as dizziness, palpitations, dyspnea, chest pain, weakness, confusion, loss of consciousness
- Previous incidence of falls
- Past medical history
- Medications taken, including alcohol use

Evaluation: History for Erectile Dysfunction

INSTRUCTIONS FOR CANDIDATE

Mr. Gupta is 54 years old and is the owner of a small business that recently failed. He has Type II diabetes and 2 years ago suffered a mild heart attack. Today, he has come to your office to discuss a problem he mentioned at the conclusion of his last visit. He was concerned about his difficulties obtaining an erection. Perform a directed history.

EVALUATION CRITERIA

I. **History**

  i. **Impotence**
  - ❏ Nature of Onset
  - ❏ Course and Frequency
  - ❏ Degree of Penile Tumescence
  - ❏ Duration of Erections
  - ❏ Palliating/Provoking Factors
  - ❏ Nocturnal Penile Tumescence
  - ❏ Erection with Self-Stimulation
  - ❏ Ability to Ejaculate/Achieve Orgasm

  ii. **Sexual History**
  - ❏ Orientation (hetero-, homo-, or bisexual)
  - ❏ Current Relationship(s)
  - ❏ Sexual Practices (oral, vaginal, anal)
  - ❏ Performance Anxiety
  - ❏ Patient's Expectations and Motivation for Rx
  - ❏ Discord with Current Sexual Partner(s)
  - ❏ Sexual Partner's (Partners') Expectations

  iii. **Risk Factors**
  Vascular
  - ❏ CAD RF (HTN, DM, smoking, dyslipidemia)
  - ❏ Coronary Artery Disease
  - ❏ Peripheral Vascular Disease.
  - ❏ Pelvic Trauma or Surgery

  Endocrine
  - ❏ Pituitary or Gonadal Dysfunction

  Neurological
  - ❏ Diabetes Mellitus
  - ❏ Alcoholism
  - ❏ Chronic Neurologic Disease (CVA, multiple sclerosis, spinal injury)

Psychological
❏ Affective Disorders (depression, anxiety)
❏ Relationship Difficulties

Other
❏ Penile Diseases (Peyronie's disease, priapism, voiding dysfunction)
❏ Penile or Pelvic Trauma
❏ Prostatitis

iv. PM History
❏ Medications and Illicit Drug Use (ethanol, sedatives, BP meds, etc.)
❏ Spinal Injury
❏ Radial Prostatectomy or Radiation

v. Impact of Erectile Dysfunction
❏ Loss of Self-Image/Self-Esteem/Self-Confidence
❏ Anxiety with Sexual Performance or Rejection
❏ Tension with Sexual Partner(s)
❏ Diminished Willingness to Initiate Sexual Relationships
❏ Withdrawal from Relationship(s)

POST-ENCOUNTER PROBES

Q1. Define impotence.
A persistent inability to obtain or sustain an adequate erection for intercourse

Q2. a. Sildenafil citrate (Viagra) is a new drug used to treat impotence. What heart medication must one ask about in the history that absolutely contraindicates the use of sildenafil?
Any nitrate drug, e.g., nitroglycerin

b. What are the relative contraindications for use of sildenafil?
Active CAD, CHF with borderline low blood pressure, concomitant use of other drugs that prolong sildenafil metabolism (e.g., cimetidine), multidrug antihypertensive regimes

c. In patients with known cardiovascular disease, which investigation should be completed before use of sildenafil?
A stress test. A patient should be able to complete >5 mets of work to tolerate sexual intercourse with his monogamous partner (roughly the same energy needed to walk up two flights of stairs). More energy is needed with new sexual partners.

Q3. a. Characterize the "typical" patient who has organic erectile dysfunction.

Older age (>50 years), persistent difficulty, risk factors (atherosclerosis, hypertension, diabetes mellitus), and absence of nocturnal penile tumescence

b. Characterize the "typical" patient who has psychogenic erectile dysfunction.

Younger age, intermittent difficulty, few to no risk factors for organic disease, nocturnal penile tumescence present, and can usually achieve erection with self-stimulation

Q4. What lab investigations would you order to narrow the cause of erectile dysfunction?

Testosterone, luteinizing hormone, follicle-stimulating hormone, prolactin, CBC, urinalysis, Cr, lipid profile, fasting blood sugar, and thyroid function studies

Q5. Name six types of drugs that are associated with impotence.

Antihypertensives, diuretics, tranquilizers, tricyclic antidepressants, serotonin reuptake inhibitors, H2-receptor antagonists, antiandrogens, alcohol, cocaine, amphetamines, and tobacco

Evaluation: History for Failure to Thrive

INSTRUCTIONS FOR CANDIDATE

Olympia Kropolous is the mother of a 3-month-old girl and is concerned about her daughter's growth. Perform a directed history.

EVALUATION CRITERIA

I. **History**

   i. **Timing**
- ❏ Since birth
- ❏ After birth

   ii. **Diet and Feeding**
- ❏ Timing and Number of Feedings
- ❏ Setting and Environment of Feedings
- ❏ Facilitation of Feedings
- ❏ Breast or Formula Feeding
- ❏ Problems with Suckling
- ❏ Position and Placement of Infant for Feeding
- ❏ Introduction of Solids
- ❏ Stooling/Vomiting Patterns Associated with Feeding

   iii. **Past Medical History**
Gestational
- ❏ Maternal Infections
- ❏ Alcohol/Substance Abuse/Smoking
- ❏ Hypertension

Perinatal
- ❏ Gestational Age (term, premature)
- ❏ Method of Delivery
- ❏ Birth Weight and Apgar Scores
- ❏ Maternal Infection

Postnatal
- ❏ Postpartum Blues/Depression
- ❏ Support System
- ❏ Developmental Milestones/Delays

Behaviour
- ❏ Infant Temperament
- ❏ Infant's Daily Routine

   iv. **Caretaker**
- ❏ Financial Concerns

❏	Other Parental Stressors
❏	Dysfunctional Marital Relationship
❏	Child-Rearing Beliefs
❏	Former Childhood Abuse or Neglect

v. Screens for Organic Causes of FTT

❏	Inadequate Intake
❏	Inadequate Absorption
❏	Poor Utilization of Nutrients
❏	Increased Energy Usage

POST-ENCOUNTER PROBES

Q1. What are the criteria for failure to thrive?

- A child younger than 2 years of age whose weight is below the 3rd or 5th percentile for age on more than one occasion OR
- A child younger than 2 years of age whose weight is less than 80% of the ideal weight for age OR
- A child younger than 2 years of age whose weight crosses two major percentiles downward on a standardized growth grid, using the 90th, 75th, 50th, 25th, 10th, and 5th percentiles as the major percentiles

Q2. What are the differential diagnoses for organic verse nonorganic FTT?

DDx Organic FTT:

- **Inadequate Intake** — insufficient breast milk, inappropriate feeding technique, cleft palate, hypotonia, lead toxicity, hypothyroidism
- **Inadequate Absorption** — celiac disease, cystic fibrosis, pancreatic insufficiency, milk allergy, inflammatory bowel disease, GI obstruction, CNS problems
- **Poor Utilization of Nutrients** — renal disease, chronic diarrhea, vomiting, diabetes mellitus and insipidus, inborn errors of metabolism
- **Increased Energy Usage** — pulmonary disease, cyanotic heart disease, chronic infections, hyperthyroidism, hypopituitarism, malignancies, juvenile rheumatoid arthritis, cerebral palsy
- **Prenatal Factors** — intrauterine infection, maternal smoking or malnutrition, fetal alcohol disorder, chromosomal disorders, hydantoin syndrome

DDx Nonorganic FTT — maternal depression, economic deprivation, emotional deprivation, dysfunctional home, child neglect/abuse, poor feeding technique, picky/poor eater, poor parent–child interaction, insufficient lactation, odd dietary beliefs and restrictions

Q3. What labs would you order to investigate FTT?

Labs are ordered only if the history and/or physical examination demonstrate a potential organic cause of FTT. They include: CBC, blood smear, electrolytes,

Ca, Mg, P, urea, creatinine, albumin, ferritin, ESR, T4, TSH, urinalysis, bone age x-ray, karyotype, immunoglobulins, sweat chloride, fecal fat.

Q4. a. Compare and contrast each of the following diagnoses: Familial Short Stature (FSS) and Constitutional Growth Delay (CGD).

FSS — Genetic background predisposes those affected to have a shorter stature. Their parents typically fall in the lower-third percentile of adult heights. They grow more slowly in the first 3 years of life but catch up to normal growth rates. Their bone age is equal to their chronological age and their weight-to-height ratios are proportional. If the child's calculated mid-parental height and the parents' heights are both in the lower-third percentile, then FSS in the absence of organic disease is the likely diagnosis.

CGD ("late bloomers") — These children decelerate in growth in the first two years, then experience growth acceleration and catch up to their peers in adolescence. Bone age is less than chronological age, and often there is a weight deficit for length.

b. How do you calculate the mid-parental heights (MPH) for males and females?

Male MPH = (father's + mother's height + 13 cm [5 in]) ÷ 2
Female MPH = (father's + mother's height − 13 cm [5 in]) ÷ 2

Q5. Give the five steps of managing a pediatric patient diagnosed with FTT.

i.   Determine and treat the underlying etiology of FTT.
ii. Institute nutritional therapy.
iii. Achieve ideal weight for height.
iv. Achieve catch-up growth.
v.   Restore optimal body composition.

Q6. Give five suggestions to the parents of a child with FTT regarding proper feeding.

i.   Eat three meals a day with at least three high-calorie snacks a day.
ii. Consume foods from each of the four food groups.
iii. Eat in a comfortable, stress-reduced environment and promote healthy eating with positive reinforcement.
iv. Offer solids first and limit liquids while ensuring adequate fluid intake.
v.   Educate parents about nutrition in children.

Evaluation: History for Fever

INSTRUCTIONS FOR CANDIDATE

Sam Wong is a 22-year-old man who presents to your practice and is concerned about a fever which he has had for the past week. Perform a directed history.

EVALUATION CRITERIA

I. **History**

   i. **Fever**

- ❑ Timing (duration, onset, and course)
- ❑ Frequency
- ❑ Quantity (What was temperature? How was it taken?)
- ❑ Aggravating/Alleviating Factors

  ii. **Associated Symptoms**

Constitutional Symptoms

- ❑ Chills/Seizures
- ❑ Night Sweats
- ❑ Weight Loss
- ❑ Change in Appetite
- ❑ Change in Sleep
- ❑ Change in Energy Level

Head and Neck Symptoms

- ❑ Headache
- ❑ Discharge from Eyes and/or Nose
- ❑ Sinus Pain
- ❑ Mouth Lesions
- ❑ Throat Pain
- ❑ Swollen Nodes

Respiratory Symptoms

- ❑ Cough
- ❑ Dyspnea/Orthopnea
- ❑ Sputum (amount, colour, blood)

Gastrointestinal Symptoms

- ❑ Nausea
- ❑ Vomiting (amount, timing, blood)
- ❑ Diarrhea (amount, timing, blood)
- ❑ Abdominal Pain (location, quality, palliating/provoking)

Neurological Symptoms
- ❏ Personality Changes/Irritability
- ❏ Lethargy/Unresponsiveness
- ❏ Loss of Consciousness
- ❏ Seizures

Musculoskeletal Symptoms
- ❏ Arthralgia (Which joints?)
- ❏ Myalgia (Which muscles?)

Skin Symptoms
- ❏ Rash (localized vs general, description, timing)
- ❏ Open Lesions (burns, bites, abrasions, foreign body)

iii. Risk Factors
- ❏ Travel History
- ❏ Infectious Contacts (children, friends, family)
- ❏ Food Poisoning (seafood, uncooked meat, fruit/vegetables)
- ❏ Contaminated Water (well/untreated water)
- ❏ Animal Contact (pets, farm, wild)
- ❏ Implanted Devices (heart valves, artificial joints, IV, saline locks, catheters)
- ❏ Immunosuppression (congenital, AIDS, co-morbid illnesses, meds)
- ❏ Vaccination Status (MMR, DPTP, HiB, Hep B, flu, TB)

II. Process Evaluation*
i. Interpersonal Skills
- ❏ Was aware of patient's nonverbal cues and emotional content
- ❏ Used reflection, checked accuracy of understanding

ii. Information Gathering
- ❏ Asked one question at a time and avoided jargon
- ❏ Used both open-ended and directed questions
- ❏ Clarified and summarized appropriately
- ❏ Ensured that patient understood questions asked
- ❏ Ensured that patient's concerns were addressed and closed interview

*See Global Process Evaluation Criteria (page 10) for a complete evaluation of the interview process.

POST-ENCOUNTER PROBES

Q1. Other than infections, what pathologies can cause fever?

Neoplastic — benign neoplasms (atrial myxoma); malignant neoplasms (lymphoma, leukemias, metastatic and solid tumours)

Inflammatory — IBD, connective-tissue diseases

Congenital — familial Mediterranean fever

Vascular — pulmonary emboli

Iatrogenic — drug-induced (malignant hypertrophy)

Q2. a. What normal physiologic event in very young children may cause a slight elevation in temperature?

Teething

> **b. What normal physiologic process will increase body temperature by as much as 0.5°C?**

Ovulation

Q3. a. Fever is often treated with antipyretics such as ASA. However, a clinician must be aware of which syndrome caused by the use of ASA in a child sick with fever?

Reye's syndrome

> **b. What two illnesses are often associated with this syndrome and the use of ASA?**

Chicken pox and influenza

> **c. What are the clinical sequelae of this syndrome?**

Lethargy, stupor, confusion, with recurrent vomiting 1 week after febrile illness. Patient may become comatose or die due to intracranial hypertension, cerebral edema, and herniation.

Evaluation: History for Gay and Lesbian Health Issues

INSTRUCTIONS FOR CANDIDATE

Damien Wallice is a 27-year-old man whom you have been following for the last 3 months in your practice as a family doctor in a rural town. At the conclusion of his last appointment, he disclosed to you that he thinks he might be gay. He has returned today to discuss these concerns. Perform a directed history.

EVALUATION CRITERIA

[Emphasize confidentiality]

I. **Development of Homosexual Identity**
  i. **Identity Confusion**
- ❑ Same-Sex Arousal
- ❑ Opposite-Sex Arousal
- ❑ Ideas, Attitudes, and Emotions about Same-Sex Couples
- ❑ Confusion

  ii. **Identity Assumption**
- ❑ Rewarding Contacts with Other Same-Sex Partners
- ❑ Self-Definition as Homosexual
- ❑ Identity Tolerance and Acceptance
- ❑ Same-Sex Sexual Exploration

  iii. **Commitment**
- ❑ Adoption of Homosexual Lifestyle
- ❑ Satisfaction with Homosexual Identity
- ❑ Commitment to a Same-Sex Relationship
- ❑ Disclosure of Sexual Identity to Heterosexuals

II. **Negative Impact of Homosexual Lifestyle**
- ❑ Level of Isolation
- ❑ Alienation from Friends and Family
- ❑ Discrimination in Education and/or Career
- ❑ Stigmatization due to HIV/AIDS
- ❑ Physical, Sexual, or Emotional Abuse by Partner(s)
- ❑ Physical, Sexual, or Emotional Abuse by Others
- ❑ Assault and Safety Issues (e.g., gay-bashing)
- ❑ History of Prostitution
- ❑ Anxiety, Depression, or Suicide
- ❑ Substance Abuse
- ❑ Eating Disorder

III. Future Relationship Goals
❏   Marriage
❏   Parenting

POST-ENCOUNTER PROBES

Q1. Identify 10 diseases for which gay men are at increased risk.

Gastrointestinal infections (*Giardia, Entamoeba, Shigella, Campylobacter,* hepatitis A), sexually transmitted diseases, HIV, hepatitis B virus, diseases from anal receptive sex (proctitis, enteritis, colitis, proctocolitis, anal syphilis, urethritis, perineal condylomata, anal fissures/fistulas), pharyngitis, substance abuse, and eating disorder

Q2. Identify some signs of confusion related to sexual orientation in adolescents.

Depression, suicidal ideation, alcohol or substance abuse, and diminished school performance

Q3. a. What is the cancer for which gay men are at elevated risk?

Anal cancer

   b. What causes this cancer?

Human Papilloma Virus

Q4. Give eight suggestions on how physicians can make their services more accessible for gays and lesbians.

Listen, never assume, be supportive, eliminate homophobic attitudes, remove judgmental attitudes, guarantee confidentiality, recognize nontraditional families, learn about health care needs of gays and lesbians, avoid referrals to homophobic health care providers.

Evaluation: History for Headache

INSTRUCTIONS FOR CANDIDATE

Sally Garat, an 18-year-old, is at a walk-in clinic where you are doing a locum. Today she is very concerned about her headache. Perform a directed history.

EVALUATION CRITERIA

I. **History**

   i. **Characteristics of Pain**
   - ❏ Location
   - ❏   Unilateral
   - ❏   Bilateral
   - ❏ Retro-orbital/Temporal/Sinus
   - ❏ Duration (hours vs days)
   - ❏ Onset (gradual vs sudden)
   - ❏ Course
   - ❏ Character (throbbing, stabbing, pressure, band-like, etc.)
   - ❏ Provoking Factors (foods [chocolate, alcohol, wine, cheese], menses, fatigue, nitrates/MSG)
   - ❏ Palliating Factors (pain meds, rest, darkness)
   - ❏ Number of Attacks

   ii. **Associated Symptoms**
   - ❏ Temporal or Sinus Tenderness
   - ❏ Lacrimation
   - ❏ Facial Flushing
   - ❏ Prodrome (scintillating scotoma, teichopsia, motor/sensory disturbance)
   - ❏ Seizures
   - ❏ Meningismus (neck pain or rigidity)
   - ❏ Increased Intracranial Pressure (nausea, vomiting, photophobia)
   - ❏ Focal Neurological Deficits (weakness, paresthesia, diplopia)
   - ❏ General Neurological Deficits (presyncope, syncope)
   - ❏ Constitutional (fever, chills, night sweats, weight loss)
   - ❏ Psychological (decr. sleep, concentration, energy, anhedonia)

   iii. **Medical History**
   - ❏ Head Trauma
   - ❏ Migraines, Pressure, or Cluster Headaches
   - ❏ Car Sickness

   iv. **Family History**
   - ❏ Migraines

POST-ENCOUNTER PROBES

Q1. What is the differential diagnosis of headache?

Migraine, cluster headaches, tension headaches, meningitis, subarachnoid/subdural/epidural hemorrhage, temporal arteritis, tumour, abscess, disease of ears/eyes/nose/sinuses/teeth/jaw/temporal mandibular joint or c-spine

Q2. a. What are the criteria for diagnosing migraines without aura?

A diagnosis of migraines without aura requires each of the following:
- Minimum of 5 attacks
- Duration of headache is 2–72 h (with or without therapy)
- Two of the following are present: unilateral pain, pulsing or throbbing quality to pain, moderate-to-severe intensity preventing daily activities, or pain provoked by routine physical activity
- One of the following is present: nausea, vomiting, photophobia, phonophobia, or osmophobia
- No evidence of other causes of headache

b. What are the criteria for diagnosing migraines with aura?

A diagnosis of migraines with aura requires all of the above plus:
- Neurological dysfunction sensed before or during attack.

Q3. Identify six ominous clinical features in a patient with headache.

i. Worst headache of the patient's life, especially if rapid onset
ii. Exacerbation of headache with coughing, sneezing, or bending down
iii. Headache with seizures, reduced level of consciousness, confusion, focal neurological findings
iv. New or progressive headache persisting for days
v. New-onset headache in middle age or older
vi. Change in the frequency, severity, or clinical features of the usual headache pattern
vii. Presence of systemic symptoms including fever, myalgia, malaise, weight loss, scalp tenderness, or jaw claudication

Q4. a. What features in the history and physical examination would increase your suspicion of temporal arteritis?

Jaw claudication, diplopia, beaded or enlarged temporal artery

b. What investigation would increase your suspicion of temporal arteritis?

Erythrocyte sedimentation rate (ESR) is abnormal (normal ESR in males is age $\div$ 2 and in females is [age + 10] $\div$ 2).

Q5. Classify the severity of migraine headaches and recommend a corresponding treatment for each level of severity.

Mild Attack — no impairment of functioning. Use ASA, ibuprofen, or acetaminophen, and possibly adjunctive therapy including dimenhydrinate, domperidone, and metoclopramide.

Moderate Attack — moderate impairment of functioning. Use ibuprofen, naproxen, mefenamic acid, sumatriptan, or dihydroergotamine.

Severe Attack — unable to function in normal activities. Use chlorpromazine, dexamethasone, sumatriptan, dihydroergotamine, metoclopramide, meperidine, or ketorolac.

Ultra-Severe Attack (status migrainus) — severe impairment >72h. Use treatment as in severe attack.

Evaluation: History for HIV

INSTRUCTIONS FOR CANDIDATE

As the medical clerk doing a rotation with a travel clinic, you are asked to see Ebion Laurent. Mr. Laurent is a 23-year-old man who has been working on board a Caribbean cruise ship as a bartender for the past 6 months. He has been referred to the clinic by his family doctor for a febrile illness and arthralgias a week after his return home. Of note were the family doctor's concerns about the patient's unprotected sexual encounters while abroad. Perform a directed history.

EVALUATION CRITERIA

I. **History**

   i. **Signs and Symptoms**
   - ❏ Flu-like Prodrome (fever, sore throat, skin rash, myalgia, arthritis)
   - ❏ AIDS (fever, night sweats, weight loss, anorexia, muscle weakness)

   ii. **Sexual History**
   - ❏ Sexually Active
   - ❏ Orientation (hetero-, homo-, or bisexual)
   - ❏ Dating and Past Relationship(s)
   - ❏ Number of Past Sexual Partners
   - ❏ Current Relationship(s)
   - ❏ Number of Current Sexual Partners
   - ❏ Sexual Practices (oral, vaginal, anal)
   - ❏ Safe Practices and Contraception (frequency of use, types)
   - ❏ Awareness of HIV/AIDS/STDs

   iii. **HIV History**
   - ❏ Previous HIV Tests (when, how many, results)
   - ❏ Last HIV Test (when; last lab results)
   - ❏ Past and Current Viral Loads and CD4+ Cell Counts (if previously HIV positive)
   - ❏ Risk Factors:
   - ❏ Contaminated Blood/Blood Products
   - ❏ Contaminated Piercings/Tattoos
   - ❏ IV Drug Use
   - ❏ Occupational Exposure
   - ❏ Organ Transplantation
   - ❏ Vertical Transmission

iv. **Medical History**
- ❏ Viral Illnesses (herpes 1&2, VZV, hepatitis B&C, HPV)
- ❏ Bacterial Illnesses (TB, syphilis)
- ❏ Last Pap Smear/Vaginal Candidiasis
- ❏ Immunization Status (tetanus, diphtheria, flu, hepatitis A/B)
- ❏ HIV Medications (current and previous meds, complications)
- ❏ Other Medications
- ❏ Drug Allergies

v. **Social History**
- ❏ Living Conditions
- ❏ Social Supports
- ❏ Employment Status
- ❏ Financial Status

II. **Process Evaluation***
   i. **Interpersonal Skills**
- ❏ Was aware of patient's nonverbal cues and emotional content
- ❏ Used reflection, checked accuracy of understanding

   ii. **Information Gathering**
- ❏ Asked one question at a time and avoided jargon
- ❏ Used both open-ended and directed questions
- ❏ Clarified and summarized appropriately
- ❏ Ensured that patient understood questions asked
- ❏ Ensured that patient's concerns were addressed and closed interview

*See Global Process Evaluation Criteria (page 10) for a complete evaluation of the interview process.

POST-ENCOUNTER PROBES

Q1. Provide four criteria that would confirm a diagnosis of acquired immunodeficiency syndrome in an HIV patient.

i.   CD4 <200.
ii. Usual AIDS-defining illness
iii. Cervical cancer
iv. Pulmonary TB
v.   Recurrent pneumonia >2/year

Q2. What investigations should be ordered for a patient who has recently been diagnosed as HIV positive?

CBC, CD4+ counts, BUN, Cr, liver transaminases (ALT/AST/ALP/LDH/GGT), protein and albumin, lipid profile, HIV viral load, VRDL, HBsAg and anti-HBs, TB skin test, Pap smear, C&S for vaginal yeast, chest x-ray (+/– pulmonary function tests)

Q3. HIV patients are at risk for various opportunistic infections at different CD4+ levels. Identify four opportunistic infections, their corresponding CD4+ levels, and their appropriate treatments.

i.   **Any CD4 Level** — Tuberculosis
     Rx — INH (9 months) or rifampin + pyrizinamide (2 months)

ii. **Any CD4 Level** — *Pneumococcus*
     Rx — vaccination

iii. **Any CD4 Level** — hepatitis A and B
     Rx — vaccination

iv. **CD4 <200** — *Pneumocystis carinii* pneumonia + oral candida
     Rx — trimethoprim–sulfamethoxazole + fluconazole

v.   **CD4 <100 and IgG** — Toxoplasma
     Rx — Septra/Dapsone + folinic acid + pyrimethamine

vi. **CD4 <50** — *Mycobacterium avium-intracellulare*
     Rx — azithromycin/rifabutin/clarithromycin

Q4. Identify six different points of discussion you would pursue with a newly diagnosed HIV-positive patient in his or her initial management.

i.   Review patient's knowledge and the implications of the diagnosis.
ii. Discuss the general long-term effects of an HIV infection.
iii. Discuss the steps needed in the prophylaxis against opportunistic infections, including immunizations.
iv. Review patient's personal supports, e.g., family, friends, co-workers.
v.   Discuss the need for reducing high-risk behaviours that could potentiate the spread of HIV to others or allow the patient to become re-infected.
vi. Discuss the need for telling sexual contacts.
vii. Outline both short-term and long-term treatment goals, including the necessity for initial investigations.

Evaluation: Management of Hypertension

INSTRUCTIONS FOR CANDIDATE

Complete a discussion with Victoria Hurley, a middle-aged patient newly diagnosed with essential hypertension. Include a brief discussion concerning a management plan for her hypertension and discuss its potential complications.

EVALUATION CRITERIA

I. History

    i. History of Hypertension
- [ ] Time Course with Elevated BPs

    ii. End-Organ Damage
- [ ] Angina or MI
- [ ] TIA/Stroke
- [ ] Peripheral Vascular Disease
- [ ] Kidney Disease

    iii. Risk Factor Assessment
- [ ] Age
- [ ] Male/Postmenopausal Female
- [ ] Smoking
- [ ] Diabetes
- [ ] Hyperlipidemia/Hypercholesterolemia
- [ ] Hyperhomocysteinemia
- [ ] FHx CAD/Strokes/PVD
- [ ] Past Medical Conditions and Medications

II. Therapeutic Discussion

    i. Risk Factor Modification
- [ ] Smoking Cessation
- [ ] Alcohol Restriction
- [ ] Weight Reduction

    ii. Dietary Modification
- [ ] Salt Restriction
- [ ] Reduction in Saturated Fat Intake

    iii. Lifestyle Alterations
- [ ] Need for Moderate Level of Exercise
- [ ] Stress Management/Modifications

    iv. Pharmacologic Therapy
- [ ] BP meds (type, dosing, complications, follow-up)

POST-ENCOUNTER PROBE

Q1. Identify 10 causes of secondary hypertension.

Renal — renal parenchymal disease (glomerulonephritis, polycystic disease, diabetic nephropathy)

Endocrine — hypo- or hyperthyroidism, pheochromocytoma, Cushing's syndrome, Conn's syndrome, hyperparathyroidism, hypercalcemia

Neurologic — brain tumour, spinal cord trauma, sleep apnea, porphyria

Toxic — alcohol, cocaine, lead poisoning, oral contraceptives, hormone replacement therapy, NSAIDs, ephedrine, corticosteroids, monoamine oxidase inhibitors

Other — aortic coarctation, pregnancy, carcinoid syndrome, pain, anxiety, hypoglycemia, alcohol or drug withdrawal

Q2. List all the routine investigations you would carry out with all newly diagnosed hypertensive patients.

Urinalysis, CBC, electrolytes, BUN, creatinine, fasting glucose and lipid profiles, EKG

Q3. Provide five nonpharmacologic therapies to reduce blood pressure in hypertensive patients.

i.   Assessment of body mass index (BMI). If BMI >25, then reduce weight by at least 4.5 kg, but weight loss to a BMI between 18 and 25 is preferred
ii. Limiting alcohol consumption to a maximum of 2 standard drinks per day for a total of 14 drinks per week for males or 9 drinks per week for females
iii. Telling hypertensive patients they should exercise 3–4 times per week at a moderate level of intensity for 50–60 minutes
iv. Restricting salt to 90–130 mmol or 3–7 g per day
v.   Smoking cessation
vi. Stress management

Q4. a. Define accelerated hypertension.

Asymptomatic; systolic BP >200 mmHg +/– diastolic BP >120 mmHg

b. Why is this a concern?

This blood pressure needs immediate therapy to prevent potential complications of a malignant hypertensive crisis.

Q5. a. How is malignant hypertension defined?

Symptomatic accelerated hypertension, the manifestations of which can include papilledema, bulging discs, retinal hemorrhages, mental status changes, and elevated creatinine

b. Identify seven associated complications of a malignant hypertensive emergency.

Confusion, seizures, headaches, visual changes, cerebral thrombosis, intracerebral or subarachnoid hemorrhage, unstable angina, myocardial infarction, acute pulmonary edema, dissecting aortic aneurysm, severe pre-eclampsia and eclampsia, acute renal failure, and pheochromocytoma

Evaluation: History for Insomnia

INSTRUCTIONS FOR CANDIDATE

François LeBlanc is a 42-year-old man whom you have followed for years in your practice. Today he presents with trouble sleeping for the last month. Perform a directed history.

EVALUATION CRITERIA

I. **History**

i. **Insomnia**
- ❏ Initial Onset of Insomnia
- ❏ Duration of Insomnia
- ❏ Quality (intermittent or continuous)
- ❏ Quantity (number of sleepless nights/week)
- ❏ Course (increasing or decreasing)
- ❏ Aggravating/Alleviating Factors
- ❏ Impact of Insomnia (work, recreation, social activities)
- ❏ Patient's Idea of Causation
- ❏ Actions Taken by Patient
- ❏ Timing of Daily Sleep Disturbance
- ❏ Trouble with Falling Asleep
- ❏ Trouble Staying Asleep
- ❏ Trouble with Early-Morning Waking

ii. **Sleep Habits**
- ❏ Time of Retiring/Awakening
- ❏ Time Taken to Fall Asleep/Wake Up
- ❏ Total Duration of Sleep
- ❏ Frequency of Awakenings
- ❏ Number of Naps in the Day

iii. **Before-Sleep Onset**
- ❏ Activities Done (e.g., strenuous exercise)
- ❏ Anxieties/Worrisome Thoughts
- ❏ Bodily Tension
- ❏ Symptoms Preventing Sleep (e.g., pain)
- ❏ Sleep Environment
- ❏ Use of Medications
- ❏ Use of Recreational Drugs
- ❏ Use of Caffeine/Nicotine/Alcohol

iv. **Sleep Period**
- ❏ Etiologies of Interruption:

- ❏ Nocturia
- ❏ Pain
- ❏ Orthopnea/Dyspnea
- ❏ Emotions During Sleep Interruption (e.g., sadness, despondency, anger)

   v. Sleep Conclusion/Awaking
- ❏ Symptoms (pain, headache)
- ❏ Emotional State

POST-ENCOUNTER PROBE

Q1. Provide a differential diagnosis of a patient having trouble with initiating or maintaining sleep.

- Transient Stress Reactions or Adjustment Reactions
- Psychiatric Disorders (depression, anxiety)
- Restless Legs Syndrome
- Psychophysiologic Insomnia
- Drug and/or Alcohol Abuse
- Disturbances of Sleep–Wake Cycle
- Sleep-Related Respiratory Disorders

Q2. What is the differential diagnosis of a patient having trouble with maintaining wakefulness?

- Sleep-Related Respiratory Disorder
- Sleep Deprivation (voluntary/enforced)
- Narcolepsy
- Drug and/or Alcohol Withdrawal
- Disturbances of Circadian Sleep–Wake Cycle
- Psychiatric Disorders
- Restless Legs Syndrome

Q3. a. Name 10 medical conditions that cause sleep disruption related to pain.

Headache — migraines, cluster headaches, head injuries, tumours

CVS — angina, MI

GI — hunger, reflux disease, duodenal ulcer

GU — menstrual pain, renal colic, UTI

MSK — mechanical neck/back strains, arthritis, gout, nocturnal leg cramps

   b. Name eight medical conditions that cause sleep disruption unrelated to pain.

Nocturia — age-related, infection-related, related to prostatic/bladder tumours

Endocrine — diabetes, hyperthyroidism, hypocalcemia, allergies, asthma, drugs

Q4. List 10 suggestions to promote better sleep hygiene.

i.   Avoid stimulating behaviour before sleep.
ii.   Do not go to bed until drowsy.
iii.   Get up at the same time every morning.
iv.   Do not nap during the day.
v.   Do not consume alcohol within 2 hours of bedtime.
vi.   Do not consume caffeine after 4 p.m.
vii.   Reduce (preferably eliminate) smoking, especially within 4 hours of bedtime.
viii. Exercise regularly before 6 p.m.
ix.   A light carbohydrate snack may promote sleep.
x.   Promote comfort while minimizing noise and light levels in the sleep environment.

Q5. Name eight common drugs that could affect sleep.

Alcohol or its withdrawal, anticonvulsants, appetite suppressants, benzodiazepine withdrawal, caffeine, diuretics, nicotine, theophylline, thyroxine, bronchodilators

Evaluation: History for Menorrhagia

INSTRUCTIONS FOR CANDIDATE

Maria Fernandez is a 42-year-old female complaining of heavy vaginal bleeding for 2 months. She is otherwise in good health. Perform a directed history.

EVALUATION CRITERIA

I.   **History**

   i.   **Vaginal Bleeding and Menses**
- ❏ Duration of Bleeding
- ❏ Frequency of Bleeding
- ❏ Postcoital Bleeding
- ❏ Severity and Quantity of Bleeding (no. of pads/day)
- ❏ Duration, Frequency, and Regularity of Menses
- ❏ Last Menses

   ii. **Obstetric and Gynecologic**
- ❏ Pregnancy (nausea, vomiting, breast pain, urinary frequency, fatigue)
- ❏ Pelvic Pain/Pressure
- ❏ Dyspareunia

   iii. **Endocrine (Screen for symptoms of)**
- ❏ Hypothyroidism (cool, dry skin; cold intolerance, constipation, fatigue)
- ❏ Prolactinoma (galactorrhea, visual changes, headache)
- ❏ Hyperandrogenism (acne, hirsutism, temporal balding, deepening of voice)
- ❏ Hypothalamic Dysfunction (anorexia, excessive exercise, stress)

   iv. **Anemia**
- ❏ Headache
- ❏ Weakness
- ❏ Presyncope
- ❏ Chest Pain

   v.   **Past Medical History**
- ❏ Coagulopathy
- ❏ Current Illnesses
- ❏ Current Medications

POST-ENCOUNTER PROBES

Q1. a. What would you order to investigate anovulatory uterine bleeding?

ß-HCG, TSH, prolactin, day 21–23 17-OH progesterone, FSH, LH, androgens, coagulation profiles, CBC, transvaginal ultrasound, sonohysterography, endometrial sampling

b. When is endometrial biopsy appropriate to order?

Age >35 years; those at high risk for endometrial hyperplasia (nulliparous 2° to infertility, heavy irregular bleeding, weight >90 kg, polycystic ovarian disease, family Hx of endometrial or colonic cancer)

Q2. What is the acute hormonal treatment of uterine bleeding?

Premarin 25 mg IV q4h x 4 doses plus Gravol to treat nausea and vomiting. Next, start levonorgestrel or norethindrone acetate 2 pills OD x 1–3 weeks.

Q3. What is the differential diagnosis of:

a. anatomic,

Anatomic — neoplasms of the vulva, vagina, or cervix; fibroids, intrauterine polyp, endometrial hyperplasia/carcinoma, coagulopathies

b. ovulatory, and

Ovulatory — abnormal prostaglandin metabolism, excessive fibrinolytic activity, congenital or acquired coagulopathy

c. anovulatory vaginal bleeding?

Anovulatory — immature hypothalamic-pituitary-ovarian axis, hypothalamic dysfunction (anorexia, excessive exercise, anorexia/bulimia), hyperprolactinemia, hypothyroidism, hyperandrogenism (polycystic ovarian disease), premature ovarian failure, menopause

Q4. What are the medical treatment options for a patient with:

a. ovulatory menorrhagia?

NSAIDs, tranexamic acid, combined OCP, danazol

b. anovulatory menorrhagia?

Clomiphene citrate and weight loss (for PCOD), combined OCP, cyclical progesterone

c. What are the surgical treatments?

Dilatation and curettage, endometrial ablation, hysterectomy

Evaluation: History for Nausea and Vomiting

INSTRUCTIONS FOR CANDIDATE

You are a physician in the local emergency department where Sinjathy Koomani, a 25-year-old female, presents with both nausea and vomiting. Perform a directed history.

EVALUATION CRITERIA

I. **History**

    i. **Nausea and Vomiting**
- ❑ Timing (duration, onset, and course)
- ❑ Frequency
- ❑ Quantity
- ❑ Quality (colour, odour, feculent, bilious, blood, coffee grounds, projectile)

    ii. **Associated Symptoms**
       Constitutional Symptoms
- ❑ Fever
- ❑ Chills
- ❑ Night Sweats
- ❑ Changes in Appetite
- ❑ Weight Changes
- ❑ Sleep Changes
- ❑ Energy Level

       Other Symptoms
- ❑ Tinnitus
- ❑ Vertigo
- ❑ Dysphagia/Odynophagia
- ❑ Changes in Bowel Movements (diarrhea, constipation, blood, melena)
- ❑ Changes in Urination (dysuria, hematuria)

    iii. **Risk Factors**
- ❑ Travel History
- ❑ Infectious Contacts (children, friends, family)
- ❑ Food Poisoning (seafood, uncooked meat, fruit/vegetables)
- ❑ Contaminated Water (well/untreated water)
- ❑ Drugs (chemotherapy, oral contraceptives, antibiotics, antiarrhythmics, morphine)
- ❑ Pregnancy
- ❑ Chronic Diseases (peptic ulcer, liver disease, migraines, CNS disease)

POST-ENCOUNTER PROBES

Q1. Provide a differential diagnosis for nausea and vomiting.

GI Tract — gastroenteritis, peptic ulcer, cholecystitis, hepatitis, pancreatitis, intestinal obstruction, ileus, appendicitis volvulus

Endocrine — pregnancy

CNS — increased ICP (trauma, tumours, meningitis)

Other — myocardial ischemia, diabetic ketoacidosis, renal failure, bulimia

Medications — contraceptives, antiarrhythmics, chemotherapy, antibiotics, morphine

Q2. In a nauseated and vomiting patient, it is important to check for dehydration. Provide several ways to examine fluid status.

Postural hypotension, jugular venous pressure, dryness of mucous membranes, skin turgor, changes in weight, urine output

Q3. What are some investigations and laboratory work you would consider ordering in a 25-year-old female patient who has been vomiting for a couple of days?

CBC, electrolytes, liver function tests, amylase, lipase, pregnancy test, abdominal series, endoscopy

Q4. Provide a differential diagnosis of vomiting in a newborn.

Gastroenteritis, gastroesophageal reflux, overfeeding, food allergy, milk protein intolerance, congenital duodenal atresia, pyloric stenosis, volvulus, meconium ileus, Hirschsprung's disease

Evaluation: History for an Obstructed Bowel

INSTRUCTIONS FOR CANDIDATE

It is 2:30 a.m. and you are the only emergency physician working. A nurse in the department asks you to assess Mario Lemay, a 65-year-old man, who looks unwell and has had nausea and vomiting for 2 days. Perform a directed history.

EVALUATION CRITERIA

I. **History**

   i. **Abdominal Pain**
   - ❏ Location (localized, diffuse, radiating, referred)
   - ❏ Timing (duration, onset, course)
   - ❏ Character (quality—diffuse, crampy, or colicky)
   - ❏ Severity

   ii. **Associated Symptoms**
   - ❏ Nausea
   - ❏ Vomiting (bilious, feculent, hematemetic)
   - ❏ Jaundice
   - ❏ Dark Urine
   - ❏ Recent Weight Loss (amount, time course)

   iii. **Changes in Bowel Movements**
   - ❏ Constipation/Obstipation
   - ❏ Change in Frequency
   - ❏ Tenesmus
   - ❏ Calibre of Stool
   - ❏ Melena
   - ❏ Hemochezia
   - ❏ Flatus

   iv. **Medical History**
   - ❏ Constipation
   - ❏ Abdominal Hernia
   - ❏ Gallstones
   - ❏ Colon Cancer
   - ❏ Previous Surgeries
   - ❏ Drugs (opiates, anticholinergics, antipsychotics)

POST-ENCOUNTER PROBES

Q1. What are the findings one would expect on an abdominal plain film in a bowel-obstructed patient?

- Dilated loops of small and/or large bowel
- Air–fluid levels

Q2. a. Name seven causes of small-bowel obstruction.

Adhesions, hernias, strictures from IBD, gallstone ileus, mesenteric artery syndrome, small-bowel tumours, metastatic cancer, cystic fibrosis, volvulus, Crohn's disease

b. Name seven causes of large-bowel obstruction.

Colon cancer, volvulus, diverticulitis, ileus, narcotics ileus, mesenteric ischemia, IBD with stricture, Ogilvie's syndrome, adhesions, intussusception, endometriosis

Q3. a. What are the first four treatment measures you would institute for a person with a complete small intestinal obstruction?

i.   Correct fluid imbalances — replace half the estimated total loss in the first 8 hours and the remaining half over the next 16 hours using isotonic saline solution or lactated Ringer's solution.
ii. Correct the electrolyte imbalances — add potassium to the infusing solution when urine output has been normalized (0.5 mL/kg/h).
iii. Insert a nasogastric tube and begin intermittent suction.
iv. Use pain control as needed.
v.   Proceed with surgery to correct the small-bowel obstruction.

b. What changes in management occur if the obstruction is partial?

Can delay surgery if there is no detectable hernia or previous history of abdominal surgery, as self-resolution is possible in partial small-bowel obstruction. Investigate the potential cause of the partial obstruction with upper GI series with follow-through or abdominal CT.

c. Identify three potential complications of bowel obstruction.

Complications from an obstructed bowel include open perforation, septicemia, and hypovolemia.

Evaluation: History for Oliguria

INSTRUCTIONS FOR CANDIDATE

Brian Goldstein is a 54-year-old man who presents to you, his family physician, with a concern about changes in his urination and swollen ankles. He is troubled with osteoarthritis in his back and knees and has been taking a nonsteroidal anti-inflammatory drug for relief of his pain. He has a past medical history of hypertension. Perform a directed history.

EVALUATION CRITERIA

I. **History**

   i. **Oliguria**
- ❏ Frequency of Urination
- ❏ Am't of Urine/Void
- ❏ Hematuria
- ❏ Discharge

   ii. **Prerenal**
- ❏ Decreases in Fluid Intake
- ❏ Fluid Loss:
- ❏   Vomiting
- ❏   Diarrhea
- ❏ Nasogastric Suction
- ❏ Volume Loss (thirst, dry mucous membranes, etc.)
- ❏ Blood Loss:
- ❏   Upper and Lower Resp. Tract (copious epistaxis, hemoptysis)
- ❏   GI Tract (hematemesis, melena, hemochezia)
- ❏   GU Tract (hematuria, menorrhagia, metrorrhagia)
- ❏ Fluid Redistribution:
- ❏   CHF (chest pain, dyspnea, orthopnea, PND, presyncope)
- ❏   Sepsis
- ❏   Third Spacing (internal bleed, pancreatitis)

   iii. **Renal**
- ❏ Recent Use of Nephrotoxic Meds (aminoglycosides, contrast, NSAIDs, sulfanilamides, thiazides, rifampin, allopurinol, cimetidine, phenytoin, analgesics, chemotherapy)
- ❏ Renal Infections (constitutional symptoms, CVA pain, hematuria)
- ❏ Recent URTI (post-streptococcal glomerulonephritis)
- ❏ Systemic Infections (SLE, diabetes, etc.)

   iv. **Postrenal**
- ❏ Obstructive Symptoms (postvoid dribbling, hesitancy,

intermittence, etc.)
❏ Irritative Symptoms (constitutional symptoms, renal colic, frequency, urgency)
❏ Hx of Renal Stones, BPH, Bladder Tumour, Neurologic Trauma

POST-ENCOUNTER PROBES

Q1. a. What is the expected rate of urine production in a healthy individual?

- 0.5 cc/mL/kg for patients older than 12 years old
- 1 cc/mL/kg for patients under 12 years old

b. Define oliguria and anuria for a typical patient.

- Oliguria is characterized by a urine output of 400–500 mL/day.
- Anuria is characterized by a urine output of <100 mL/day.

Q2. What investigations would you order on admission?

CBC, electrolytes, BUN, Cr, glucose, urate, Ca^{2+}, Mg^{2+}, phosphate, blood osmolarity, ESR, urinalysis, culture and sensitivity plus routine and microscopy of urine, urine osmolarity, 24-h urine for protein, pH and osmolarity, abdominal and pelvic ultrasound, abdominal x-ray

Q3. What is the frequency of prerenal, renal, and postrenal causes of acute renal failure?

Prerenal Causes — account for approximately 70% of acute renal failure due to reductions in renal perfusion by such causes as extracellular volume loss (vomiting, diarrhea, GI hemorrhage).

Renal Causes — account for approximately 20% of acute renal failure. The most common cause is acute tubular necrosis, often due to prolonged hypoperfusion, sepsis, or nephrotoxic agents. Acute glomerulonephritis and acute interstitial nephritis are other causes of renal failure.

Postrenal Causes — account for the remaining 10% of cases. These are usually obstructive in nature. They can be subcategorized as extrarenal obstructions (prostate cancer, BPH, renal stones, bladder tumour, neurogenic bladder) or intrarenal obstructions (amyloidosis, multiple myeloma).

Q4. What are the major complications of acute renal failure?

Hyperuricemia, hyponatremia, volume expansion, CHF, hyperkalemia, arrhythmias, acidosis, hyperphosphatemia, hypocalcemia, hypermagnesemia, anemia, drug toxicities, reduced diuretic efficacy

Q5. What are the cardiovascular, pulmonary, and nervous system effects of uremic toxicity?

Cardiovascular — cardiomyopathy, arrhythmias, pericarditis, accelerated atherosclerosis

Pulmonary — pulmonary edema, pneumonitis, pleuritis

Nervous — irritability, insomnia, anorexia, seizures, coma, restless legs, foot/wrist drop, glove-and-stocking paresthesia

Evaluation: History for Oral Contraception

INSTRUCTIONS FOR CANDIDATE

Daisy Ewing is a 16-year-old who has come to your office because she wants to start taking the birth control pill. Her previous visits have been for annual check-ups and the occasional upper respiratory infection, but she last saw you 3.5 years ago. Her past medical record is otherwise unremarkable. Perform a directed history.

EVALUATION CRITERIA

I. **History**

   i. **Initial Screen**
   - ❏ Currently Sexually Active
   - ❏ Orientation (hetero-, homo-, or bisexual)
   - ❏ Dating and Past Relationship(s)
   - ❏ Number of Past Sexual Partners
   - ❏ Current Relationship(s)
   - ❏ Number of Current Sexual Partners
   - ❏ Sexual Practices (oral, vaginal, anal)
   - ❏ Safe Practices and Contraception (frequency of use, types)
   - ❏ Awareness of STDs

   ii. **Menstrual History**
   - ❏ Age of Onset
   - ❏ Length of Period
   - ❏ Regularity of Period
   - ❏ Intermenstrual Bleeding
   - ❏ Last Pap Smear Result
   - ❏ Premenstrual Syndrome

   iii. **Obstetric/Gynecologic History**
   - ❏ Previous Pregnancy(ies)
   - ❏ Previous Gynecologic Procedures

   iv. **Past Medical History**
   - ❏ Hypertension
   - ❏ Active Liver Disease
   - ❏ Thromboembolic disease
   - ❏ Migraines
   - ❏ Cancer of Breast, Ovary, Uterus, or Colon
   - ❏ Current Medications
   - ❏ Alcohol/Drug Hx
   - ❏ Hx of Smoking

POST-ENCOUNTER PROBES

Q1. Describe the five benefits of oral contraception.

i.   Pregnancy is prevented.
ii. Menses are regular, lighter, and shorter in duration.
iii. Cramping and PMS are reduced.
iv. Acne may improve.
v.   Risk of ovarian cysts and benign breast disease is reduced.

Q2. Like most medications, oral contraceptives have side effects. Identify five side effects related to:

 a. estrogen excess

Estrogen Excess — cystic breast changes, breast or uterine enlargement, mucorrhea, uterine fibroid growth, dysmenorrhea/hypermenorrhea/menorrhagia, presyncope/syncope, edema, leg cramps, nausea, vomiting, weight gain

 b. progesterone excess

Progesterone Excess — increased appetite, decreased libido, acne, hirsutism, edema, depression, cervicitis, fatigue, weight gain, hypertension

 c. estrogen deficiency

Estrogen Deficiency — nervousness, continuous bleeding, spotting in first half of cycle (days 1–9), atrophic vaginitis, urinary incontinence

 d. progesterone deficiency

Progesterone Deficiency — late menstrual bleeding (days 10–21), dysmenorrhea, heavy flow, delayed withdrawal bleed, bloating, dizziness, headache, irritability, nausea, vomiting, visual changes, weight gain

 e. androgen excess

Androgen Excess — weight gain, edema, increased libido, acne, hirsutism, oily skin and scalp, jaundice, rash, pruritus

Q3. Name eight contraindications to the use of OCP.

i.   Current Pregnancy
ii.   Undiagnosed Vaginal Bleeding
iii. Cardiovascular Disease (thromboembolic/cerebrovascular/coronary events)
iv.   Estrogen-Dependent Tumours (breast, uterus, liver)
v.   Impaired Liver Function
vi.   Congenital Hyperlipidemia
vii. Wilson's Disease
viii. Age >35 and Smoking

Q4. What drugs interact with OCPs, reducing their efficacy?

Antibiotics, anticonvulsants, and antacid

Evaluation: History for Otitis Media

INSTRUCTIONS FOR CANDIDATE

Taliya Silver Sky, an 18-month-old infant, has been brought to the emergency department by her grandmother, who is concerned about the child's irritability. Perform a directed history.

EVALUATION CRITERIA

I. **History**

   i. **Clinical Features**
   - ❏ Ear-Tugging
   - ❏ Hearing Loss
   - ❏ Loss of Balance
   - ❏ Otorrhea (discharge from ear)
   - ❏ Irritability
   - ❏ Poor Sleep
   - ❏ Anorexia
   - ❏ Vomiting
   - ❏ Diarrhea

   ii. **Past Medical History**
   - ❏ Previous OM
   - ❏ Recent URTI
   - ❏ Recent Allergies
   - ❏ Chronic Sinusitis

   iii. **Risk Factors**
   - ❏ Bottle Feeding
   - ❏ Passive Smoke
   - ❏ Day Care/Group Child Care Facilities
   - ❏ Low Socioeconomic Status
   - ❏ Craniofacial Abnormalities (e.g., cleft palate)

POST-ENCOUNTER PROBES

Q1. What is the pathogenesis of otitis media?

Otitis media is an inflammatory condition of the middle ear that is initiated by functional or mechanical obstruction of the eustachian tube leading to negative middle-ear partial pressure. Subsequently, transudation of capillary serous fluid into the middle-ear space follows. Nasopharyngeal bacteria may invade the middle-ear space via the obstructed eustachian tube and replicate within the serous middle-ear fluid. Bacterial and inflammatory host cell products are released, attracting peripheral blood leukocytes, leading to a cascade of acute inflammatory events that result in acute OM.

Q2. What is the peak age range for acute OM?

Age 3 months to 3 years (60%–70% of children have at least one episode of AOM before 3 years of age)

Q3. a. What are the three main etiologies of AOM in children?

S. pneumoniae (30%), *H. influenzae* (20%), *M. catarrhalis* (20%), viral (20%–25%), group A strep (5%)

b. What is the recommended treatment for otitis media, given the most common cause of OM in otherwise healthy patients older than 2 years and in patients 2 years old or younger?

Watchful waiting for 48 h, fluids, and pain and fever control with acetaminophen in patients older than 2 years old are recommended, as the most common cause of OM is viral. In children 2 years old or younger, fluids, acetaminophen, and amoxicillin (40 mg/kg/day x 5 days) should be used.

c. Name three conditions that should prompt immediate antibiotic therapy despite age.

Children with craniofacial abnormalities, those who are immunocompromised or malnourished, or children recently treated with antibiotics are less likely to resolve OM infections without antibiotics.

Q4. Identify three acute extra-aural complications of bacterial otitis media.

Mastoiditis, meningitis, facial nerve paralysis, and brain abscesses

Q5. What is the name of the vaccine that may lessen the burden of streptococcal infections and therefore lessen potential OM infections in children?

Prevnar—useful in 97% of children from 6 weeks to 2 years old

Q6. a. How long will a tympanic effusion take to resolve in most children?

Sixty to ninety per cent of effusions will resolve within 12 weeks.

b. What are the indications for tympanostomy tube placement?

Abnormal audiology assessment, language delays, and effusion lasting >16 weeks. Consensus regarding specific indications for tube placement with recurrent otitis media infections is lacking, but a quick rule is >5 OM infections per year or >3 OM infections per season require tube placement.

c. What are three potential long-term complications of tympanostomy tube placement?

Atrophy, retraction pockets, and perforation

Evaluation: History for Overdose

INSTRUCTIONS FOR CANDIDATE

Lance Lockhart, a 21-year-old university student, was admitted with a drug overdose. You are a member of the inpatient psychiatric team. Perform a directed history.

EVALUATION CRITERIA

I. History

i. Depression
- ❏ Weight
- ❏ Appetite Changes
- ❏ Energy Level
- ❏ Sleep Changes
- ❏ Changes in Interest in Activities and Motivation
- ❏ Changes in Libido
- ❏ Changes in Attention and Concentration
- ❏ Memory Changes
- ❏ Feelings of Guilt
- ❏ Feelings of Worthlessness

ii. Assessment for Suicidal Status
- ❏ Passive (Is life not worth living?)
- ❏ Active (Thought of taking your life?)
- ❏ Ascertaining Urgency of Attempt
- ❏ Ascertaining Plan (where, when, and how)
- ❏ Ascertaining Reason for Attempt

iii. Risk Factors for Suicide
- ❏ Depression/Schizophrenia
- ❏ Previous Attempts
- ❏ Ethanol/Drug Use
- ❏ Recent Loss (divorce, bereavement, unemployment)
- ❏ Suicide in Family
- ❏ Organized Plan
- ❏ Lack of Social Supports
- ❏ Serious Illness

iv. Assessment for Homicidal Status
- ❏ Ascertaining Probability of Attempt
- ❏ Ascertaining Reason for Attempt
- ❏ Ascertaining Plan (where, when, and how)

v. Assessment for Other Psychiatric Illness
☐   Orientation to Person, Place, and Time
☐   Delusions
☐   Anxieties/Phobias
☐   Obsessions/Compulsions
☐   Hallucinations
☐   Past Hospitalizations
☐   Past Psychiatric Illnesses

II. Process Evaluation*
i. Interpersonal Skills
☐   Was aware of patient's nonverbal cues and emotional content
☐   Used reflection, checked accuracy of understanding

ii. Information Gathering
☐   Asked one question at a time and avoided jargon
☐   Used both open-ended and directed questions
☐   Clarified and summarized appropriately
☐   Ensured that patient understood questions asked
☐   Ensured that patient's concerns were addressed and closed interview

*See Global Process Evaluation Criteria (page 10) for a complete evaluation of the interview process.

POST-ENCOUNTER PROBES

Q1. Identify five risk factors commonly associated with individuals attempting to commit suicide.

SAD PERSONS
Sex male
Age >60 years
Depression/Schizophrenia
Previous attempts
Ethanol abuse
Recent loss (divorce, bereavement, unemployment)
Suicide in family
Organized plan
No social supports
Serious illness

Q2. Suicide is often associated with psychiatric illness. Name four mental illnesses that carry a heightened degree of risk for suicide.

i.   Mood disorders (depression, bipolar disorder)
ii.   Schizophrenia
iii.   Eating disorders (anorexia nervosa, bulimia nervosa)
iv.   Substance abuse

Q3. Assume your patient had committed an act of self-harm in escalating efforts toward suicide. Identify three questions you might ask to assess the risk of suicide after deliberate self-harm.

i.   Was self-harm planned or impulsive?
ii. Were attempts made to seek help?
iii. Were precautions taken against being found?
iv. What was the level of danger or lethality of the act?
v.   Was a suicide note or will made?
vi. Is there remorse after the fact?
vii. Is there a psychiatric illness at work?

Q4. Teenagers form one group of patients that sometimes turn to suicide as a last resort to cope with problems they feel are beyond their control. Provide some questions you might ask a teenage patient in order to assess his or her wellness and to prevent smaller problems from becoming overwhelming ones.

One might inquire into the following areas of a teenager's life:

Home — living arrangements, relationship with parents, family issues, attempts at running away

Education — school attendance, areas of difficulty, suspensions, relationships with teachers and fellow students

Activities — after-school activities, sports played, employment

Drugs — types of alcohol and/or drugs used, smoking

Sexuality — dating, sexual experiences, current relationship(s), orientation, number of partners, frequency of intercourse, types of contraceptives used, STD awareness

Suicide — assess risk factors (see Q1: SAD PERSON); inquire into attempts, ideation, plans to commit

Evaluation: History for Heart Palpitations

INSTRUCTIONS FOR CANDIDATE

Tory Crown is 32 years old. She has been experiencing an odd sensation in her chest for a month. She has come to see you today at the insistence of her husband. Perform a directed history.

EVALUATION CRITERIA

I. **History**

   i. **Palpitations**
- ❑ Quality (slow vs rapid, regular vs irregular)
- ❑ Quantity (frequency of bouts)
- ❑ Duration
- ❑ Onset
- ❑ Palliating/Provoking Factors

   ii. **Associated Symptoms**
- ❑ Chest Pain
- ❑ Presyncope/Syncope
- ❑ Dyspnea/Orthopnea/PND
- ❑ Malaise/Fatigue
- ❑ Constitutional (fever/chills/night sweats)
- ❑ Diaphoresis
- ❑ Edema (ankle, sacral, crackles)
- ❑ Cough

   iii. **Symptoms of TIA/Stroke**
- ❑ Numbness/Paresthesia
- ❑ Weakness
- ❑ Visual Abnormalities
- ❑ Speech Abnormalities

   iv. **Potential Etiologies**
    Cardiac
- ❑ Pericardial (pericarditis)
- ❑ Myocardial (LVH, infarction, CHF, myxoma, ASD, amyloidosis)
- ❑ Endocardial (infarction, sick sinus, valvular—mitral valve regurgitation or stenosis, aortic valve regurgitation or stenosis)

    Pulmonary
- ❑ Obstructive (asthma, COPD)
- ❑ Infections (pneumonia)
- ❑ Vascular (pulmonary embolism)

Metabolic
- ❑ Endocrine (hyperthyroid, pheochromocytosis, hypoglycemia)

Toxins
- ❑ Sepsis
- ❑ EtOH (binge or withdrawal)
- ❑ CO Poisoning
- ❑ Stimulants (caffeine, theophylline, amphetamines, cocaine)

Other
- ❑ Electrolyte Abnormality

POST-ENCOUNTER PROBES

Q1. Describe the investigations you would order to discover the etiology of the heart palpitations.

Na^+, K^+, Mg^{2+}, CBC, BUN, Cr, LDH, CK, TSH, T4, cardiac enzymes, EKG, Echo, CXR

Q2. What are the important management issues concerning atrial fibrillation?

- **Rate Control** — managed with beta-blockers, Ca^{2+} channel blockers, or digoxin
- **Anticoagulation** — managed with heparin, then coumadin
- **Rhythm Conversion** — facilitated by either electro- or medical conversion
- **Determining Etiology** — completing investigations with appropriate follow-up

Q3. Give a differential diagnosis of bradyarrhythmias, conduction delays, irregular tachyarrhythmias, and regular tachyarrhythmias.

Bradyarrhythmias — sinus bradycardia, sick sinus syndrome, junctional and ventricular escape rhythmias

Conduction Delays — 1°, 2°, or 3° AV nodal block, fascicular block, and bundle branch block

Irregular Tachyarrhythmias — atrial fibrillation, multifactorial atrial tachycardia, atrial flutter with variable block, atrial or ventricular premature beats, ventricular fibrillation

Regular Tachyarrhythmias (narrow complex) — supraventricular tachycardia, atrial flutter, Wolfe-Parkinson-White syndrome, AV node re-entry tract

Regular Tachyarrhythmias (wide complex) — supraventricular tachycardia with aberrance or bundle branch block, ventricular tachycardia, torsades de pointes

Q4. a. When is a rhythm unstable?

An arrhythmia is unstable when a person has hypotension, dyspnea, chest pain, presyncope, or syncope.

b. What is the definitive treatment for any unstable arrhythmia?

Direct current cardioversion

Evaluation: History for Physical Abuse

INSTRUCTIONS FOR CANDIDATE

You are the intern working an evening shift at a women's walk-in clinic. A 22-year-old, six-months-pregnant woman who prefers not to give her name is anxious to see a doctor about headaches and gastrointestinal upset. Upon entering the examination room, you make note of a black eye and bruises on her forearms. Perform a directed history.

EVALUATION CRITERIA

I. **History**

   i. **Screens**

- ❏ Has your partner ever hit you?
- ❏ What happens during arguments?
- ❏ Has your partner ever ridiculed you or cut you off from other relationships with friends/family?
- ❏ Have you sought help from others in health care?

   ii. **Abuse Risk Factors**

- ❏ Weapon at Home
- ❏ Alcohol Abuse
- ❏ Previous Assault
- ❏ Geographic Isolation
- ❏ Escalating Levels of Violence
- ❏ Death and Suicide Threats
- ❏ Abuse Extending to Children

   iii. **Positive Indicators**

- ❏ Limited Eye Contact
- ❏ Vague Explanations of Injuries
- ❏ Scripted Explanations for Injuries
- ❏ Injuries Not Compatible with Explanation
- ❏ Injuries in Central Location (head, face, neck, breasts, abdomen)
- ❏ Multiple Injuries at Different Stages
- ❏ Noncompliance with Treatment Plans

   iv. **Further Inquiry and Confirmation**

- ❏ Do you feel safe?
- ❏ Do you feel you can speak freely on the telephone?
- ❏ Are you able to share in financial decisions?
- Does your spouse prevent you from:
- ❏   choosing friends?

❏   seeing family?
❏   attending activities outside your home?

   v. Other
❏   Reassured Confidentiality about Above
❏   Offered Assistance and Emergency Numbers
❏   Developed Safety Plan for Future Egress

II. Process Evaluation*
   i. Interpersonal Skills
❏   Was aware of patient's nonverbal cues and emotional content
❏   Used reflection, checked accuracy of understanding

   ii. Information Gathering
❏   Asked one question at a time and avoided jargon
❏   Used both open-ended and directed questions
❏   Clarified and summarized appropriately
❏   Ensured that patient understood questions asked
❏   Ensured that patient's concerns were addressed and closed
              interview

*See Global Process Evaluation Criteria (page 10) for a complete evaluation of the interview process.

POST-ENCOUNTER PROBES

Q1. How can one distinguish injuries from physical abuse versus accidental injuries?
Physical injuries from accidents usually involve the peripheral parts of the body while those of abuse involve central locations (head, face, neck, breasts, and abdomen).

Q2. Why do abused people stay in abusive relationships?
Commitment to relationship/marriage; the abused believes promises of the abuser; financial/cultural factors; fear

Q3. Describe the other kinds of abuse.
Sexual Abuse — forced sex, forced pornography, imposed pregnancy or abortion

Emotional Abuse — verbal attacks, name calling, often relentless

Psychological Abuse — control, isolation, threats

Financial Abuse — control of money, access, spending

Q4. Identify some characteristics of abusers.
Personality disorders, lack of empathy, low self-esteem, threatened masculinity, need for power and control, pathological jealousy, substance abuse, violence in family of origin, feeling threatened by fetus

Q5. You are an ER physician treating a patient you suspect has been abused by a partner. You need to inquire into the possibility of abuse, but the partner never leaves the patient's side in the ER. What can you do to get the information you need to confirm abuse?

Order an x-ray. Most people know they cannot accompany a patient into the x-ray room. Once the partner and patient are separated, you can ask the necessary questions and continue with the x-ray if required.

Q6. What should physicians do for a patient after disclosure of abuse?

DSM

Document abuse completely and accurately.

Support the abused patient (indicate it is not her/his fault, validate feelings).

Make a safety plan (help person gain access to shelters, legal options, etc.).

Evaluation: History for Postoperative Fever

INSTRUCTIONS FOR CANDIDATE

Jose Martinez is 46 years old, and you are seeing him two days after his cholecystectomy. His nurse was concerned about a high temperature. Perform a directed history.

EVALUATION CRITERIA

I. **History**

  i. **Pulmonary**
  - ☐ Chest Pain
  - ☐ Dyspnea/Orthopnea
  - ☐ Cough (nonproductive vs productive)
  - ☐ Hemoptysis

  ii. **Urinary**
  - ☐ Frequency
  - ☐ Urgency
  - ☐ Dysuria
  - ☐ Discharge/Cloudy Urine
  - ☐ Hematuria
  - ☐ Suprapubic Pain

  iii. **Wound(s) and Veins (IV line access)**
  - ☐ Inflammation (erythema, edema, heat)
  - ☐ Pain
  - ☐ Bleeding
  - ☐ Discharge

  iv. **Deep Venous Thrombosis**
  - ☐ Calf Pain
  - ☐ Inflammation (erythema, edema, heat)

  v. **Drugs**
  - ☐ Previous Meds
  - ☐ New Meds
  - ☐ Allergies
  - ☐ Blood Transfusions

II. **Process Evaluation***

  i. **Interpersonal Skills**
  - ☐ Was aware of patient's nonverbal cues and emotional content
  - ☐ Used reflection, checked accuracy of understanding

ii. Information Gathering

- ❏ Asked one question at a time and avoided jargon
- ❏ Used both open-ended and directed questions
- ❏ Clarified and summarized appropriately
- ❏ Ensured that patient understood questions asked
- ❏ Ensured that patient's concerns were addressed and closed interview

*See Global Process Evaluation Criteria (page 10) for a complete evaluation of the interview process.

POST-ENCOUNTER PROBES

Q1. Provide a differential diagnosis of post-op fever etiologies with their timing.

Post-Op Day 0–2 — atelectasis, aspiration pneumonia, wound infection, leakage of anastomosis

Post-Op Day $\geq$3 — UTI, wound infection, IV site infection, septic thrombophlebitis, abscess, deep vein thrombosis, pulmonary embolism

Q2. For paralytic ileus, describe:

a. clinical findings

No gas per rectum, abdominal distention, vomiting, absent bowel sounds

b. treatment

NG tube, fluid resuscitation, consideration of parenteral nutrition (if prolonged ileus)

c. timing for return of GI motility.

Should return by 48 h, small-bowel motility by 24–48 h, and colon motility by 3–5 days

Q3. Your patient is postoperative day 1, and the nursing staff reports that she has an altered sleep–wake cycle, decreased concentration, and agitation.

a. What is your diagnosis?

Delirium

b. Provide six risk factors for this condition.

Age >50 years, pre-existing cognitive dysfunction, depression, perioperative derangements, >5 prescribed medications postoperatively, use of anticholinergics preoperatively, cardiopulmonary bypass, ICU setting

Q4. *At postoperative day 5, your patient who underwent rectal surgery has a persistent spiking fever, dull rectal and abdominal pain, and diarrhea.*

 a. *What is your provisional diagnosis?*

Rectal abscess

 b. *What test(s) will confirm it?*

Ultrasound or CT scan

 c. *What is the treatment?*

Drainage of abscess; antibiotics to cover aerobic and anaerobic bacteria

Q5. *Give six strategies to reduce atelectasis.*

Incentive spirometry, minimal use of depressants, good pain control, early ambulation, deep breathing, and frequent changes in position

Evaluation: History for Preoperative Patient

INSTRUCTIONS FOR CANDIDATE

Maria Josefina Lopez is 52 years old and has come to your office for a complete preoperative check-up to assess her readiness for surgery. Perform a directed history.

EVALUATION CRITERIA

I. **History**

   i. **Pulmonary Assessment**

❑ Obstructive Disease (asthma, COPD)
❑ Restrictive Disease (pneumoconiosis, severe kyphosis)
❑ Sleep Apnea
❑ Recent Respiratory Infection
❑ Smoking Hx
❑ Assessment of Exercise Tolerance (no. flights of stairs)

   ii. **Cardiac Assessment**

❑ Hypertension
❑ Angina
❑ Myocardial Infarction(s)
❑ Thrombolytic Hx
❑ Angioplasty Hx
❑ Coronary Artery Bypass Grafting
❑ Congestive Heart Failure
❑ Systolic vs Diastolic
❑ New York Heart Class and LV Function
❑ Valvular Disease
    Arrhythmia:
❑   Type
❑   Pacemaker
❑ Peripheral Vascular Disease

   iii. **Nervous System Assessment**

❑ Upper Motor Neurons
❑ TIA/Cerebral Vascular Stroke
❑ Seizures
❑ Migraines/Headaches
❑ Spinal Trauma
❑ Lower Motor Neurons/Neuromuscular Disorders

   iv. **Gastrointestinal System Assessment**

❑ Reflux

❏   Hepatic Disease/Jaundice
❏   Renal Failure

v.   Endocrine System Assessment
❏   Diabetes Mellitus
❏   Thyroid Dysfunction

vi. Hematologic System Assessment
❏   Excessive Bleeding/Anemia

vii. Musculoskeletal System Assessment
❏   Cervical, Thoracic, and/or Lumbar Back Pain

viii. Dental Assessment
❏   Loose Teeth or Dentures

ix.   Medical History
❏   Medications
❏   Substance Use (alcohol/drug Hx)
❏   Allergies

POST-ENCOUNTER PROBES

Q1. What basic laboratory investigations would you order for this patient? Justify your reasons for these tests.

Ordering a battery of tests for every preoperative patient is wrong. Commonly, EKG, chest x-ray, CBC, electrolytes, Cr, and BUN are ordered for patients older than 50 years. Often these tests are of very low yield. However, they do give a baseline of function perioperatively. More specific tests can be completed if other co-morbidities exist.

Q2. For patients with cardiovascular conditions, list the preoperative investigations you might order.

EKG, stress test, stress thallium test, echocardiogram, Holter monitor, MUGA, and angiography

Q3. Use four major systems of the body as headings and create a table of potential physical findings you are looking for in a preoperative examination.

System	Finding
Circulatory	Heart sounds, rate, rhythm, murmurs, orthostatic BP, peripheral pulses, edema
Respiratory	Breath sounds, adventitia, pattern of breathing, chest wall morphology
Nervous	Level of consciousness, evidence of sensory or motor dysfunction

continued

System	Finding
Hepatic	Jaundice, ascites, tremor, spider nevi, herniated umbilicus, scleral icterus
Hematologic	Bruising, petechiae
Head/Neck	Neck flexion, mouth opening, TMJ immobility, dentition

Q4. Describe the potential intraoperative complication that may result from each of the following drugs: ASA, coumadin, insulin, oral hypoglycemics, beta-blockers, aminoglycosides, MAOIs, tricyclic antidepressants, and benzodiazepines.

Drug Name	Potential Intraoperative Complication
ASA	Bleeding
Coumadin	Bleeding
Insulin	Hypoglycemia
Oral Hypoglycemics	Hypoglycemia
Beta-Blockers	Bradycardia, myocardial depression, depression of normal compensatory circulatory responses
Aminoglycosides	Skeletal muscle weakness; potentiates the response to nondepolarizing muscle relaxants
MAOIs	Increased catecholamine responses, especially when sympathomimetics are used
TCAs	Same as MAOIs
Benzodiazepines	Increased tolerance to anesthetic drugs

Evaluation: History for Renal Colic

INSTRUCTIONS FOR CANDIDATE

Lachlan Dumont, a 39-year-old man, has had intermittent flank pain for 2 months. After a severe episode last night, he has come to your family medicine practice. Perform a directed history.

EVALUATION CRITERIA

I. History

i. Pain
- ❏ Location of Pain (unilateral vs bilateral, radiation to groin)
- ❏ Duration
- ❏ Course over Time
- ❏ Onset
- ❏ Course (ureteral colic from intermittent ureteral distention, constant flank pain from renal capsular distention)

ii. Irritative Urinary Symptoms
- ❏ Increased Frequency/Nocturia
- ❏ Urgency
- ❏ Dysuria

iii. Obstructive Urinary Symptoms
- ❏ Hesitancy
- ❏ Diminished Stream
- ❏ Postvoid Dribbling
- ❏ Postvoid Suprapubic Fullness

iv. Associated Symptoms
- ❏ Hematuria
- ❏ Diaphoresis
- ❏ Constitutional (fever/chills/night sweats/weight loss)
- ❏ Abdominal (nausea/vomiting)

v. Risk Factors
- ❏ Diet High in Oxalates (spinach, rhubarb, nuts, tea, cocoa)
- ❏ Calcium or Excess Vitamin C Administration
- ❏ Prolonged Immobilization
- ❏ Meds (chemotherapy, furosemide, hydrochlorothiazide, indinavir)
- ❏ Family Hx of Kidney Stones
- ❏ Inflammatory Bowel Disease
- ❏ Previous Urinary Tract Infections

POST-ENCOUNTER PROBES

Q1. Provide four potential steps in the initial treatment and diagnosis of renal colic.

i. Consider admission to hospital.
ii. Analgesic (acetaminophen with codeine/meperidine CDI/morphine + antiemetic)
iii. Antibiotics for UTI
iv. IV normal saline for volume replacement if vomiting
v. Investigations to include: CBC, electrolytes, Cr, BUN, urinalysis, R&M of urine, C&S of urine, and CT or abdominal ultrasound

Q2. What are the indications for admission of renal colic to hospital?

- Recalcitrant renal colic
- Persistent vomiting
- Fever/infection
- High-grade obstruction
- Single kidney with ureteral obstruction
- Bilateral ureteral stones

Evaluation: History for Seizures

INSTRUCTIONS FOR CANDIDATE

Hao Thien is 35 years old and is a new patient in your clinic. At her first visit, she stated she has a seizure disorder. You have asked her to return to obtain more information. Perform a directed history.

EVALUATION CRITERIA

I. **History**

    i. **Seizures**
- ❏ Age at Onset
- ❏ Timing (duration, onset, and course)
- ❏ Quantity
- ❏ Quality
- ❏ Frequency
- ❏ Aggravating/Alleviating Factors:
- ❏   Sleep Deprivation
- ❏   Drug/Alcohol Withdrawal
- ❏   TV/Strobe

    ii. **Associated Symptoms**
- ❏ Presence of Aura
- ❏ Salivation and Tongue Biting
- ❏ Cyanosis
- ❏ Incontinence
- ❏ Jacksonian March
- ❏ Automatisms (e.g., chewing, lip smacking, walking)

    iii. **Past Medical History**
- ❏ Birth Trauma
- ❏ Head Trauma
- ❏ Stroke
- ❏ CNS Infection
- ❏ Drug Use
- ❏ Family History of Seizure Disorder

POST-ENCOUNTER PROBES

Q1. Compare and contrast seizure and syncope.

Characteristic	Seizure	Syncope
Time of Onset	Day or night	Daytime
Position	Any	Upright (usually)
Onset	Sudden or brief aura	Gradual (vasodepression)
Aura	Possible specific aura	Dizziness, visual blurring, lightheadedness
Colour	Normal or cyanotic	Pallor
Autonomic Features	Uncommon	Common
Duration	Brief or prolonged	Brief
Urinary Incontinence	Sometimes	Rare
Motor Activity	Sometimes	Rare
Automatisms	Can occur	None
EEG	Frequently abnormal	Usually normal

Q2. Characterize the different types of seizure disorders.

Seizures can be partial (affecting a part of the brain) or generalized (affecting the whole brain). There are two types of partial seizures, including simple (awareness of events intact) and complex (diminished awareness of events). There are five kinds of generalized seizures, including: absence (person "phases out" into a blank stare), myoclonic (movements are quick and jerking), tonic–clonic (muscles alternate between movement and stiffness), tonic (muscles are stiff), and atonic ("drop seizures"). All generalized seizures entail diminished awareness of events. Sometimes partial seizures progress to generalized seizures.

Q3. What are some causes of seizures in:
   a. children
   b. adults
   c. the elderly?

Children — seizures are often the result of infections, trauma, metabolic or congenital and genetic abnormalities.

Adults — seizures are often the result of infections, trauma, strokes, or tumours.

Elderly — seizures are often the result of infections, trauma, strokes, tumours, or metabolic abnormalities.

Evaluation: History for Sexual Abuse

INSTRUCTIONS FOR CANDIDATE

You are the new resident on call for the psychiatric service in a large city hospital. You are called to see an 18-year-old woman whom you recognize as the stepdaughter of your next-door neighbour. She has recently moved into the apartment next to yours. You have heard heated conversations and sobbing coming from this apartment over the last month. Perform a directed history.

EVALUATION CRITERIA

I. **History**

   i. **Physical Abuse Screens**
      Did a parent or other adult in the household:
      ❏ Often push, grab, shove, or slap you?
      ❏ Often hit you, resulting in injuries or visible marks?

   ii. **Psychological Abuse Screens**
      Did a parent or other adult in the household:
      ❏ Often swear at, insult, or belittle you?
      ❏ Often act in a way that caused you to fear injury?

   iii. **Sexual Abuse Screens**
      Did a parent or other adult in the household:
      ❏ Touch or fondle you in a sexual way?
      ❏ Have you touch his or her body in a sexual way?
      ❏ Attempt or actually have oral, anal, or vaginal intercourse with you?

   iv. **Additional Abuse Screens**
      In your home, was there:
      ❏ Substance abuse?
      ❏ Mental illness?
      ❏ Abuse of other family members?
      ❏ Criminal behaviour?

   v. **Medical Consequences**
      Somatic Complaints
      ❏ Chronic Headaches/Migraines
      ❏ Pain (abdominal, pelvic, thoracic, throat) and/or IBS

      Post-traumatic Stress Disorder
      ❏ Hyperarousal
      ❏ Insomnia

- ❏ Nightmares
- ❏ Problems with Anger Management

Psychiatric Disorders
- ❏ Depression/Anxiety
- ❏ Suicidal Gestures or Attempts
- ❏ Low Self-Esteem
- ❏ Personality/Dissociative Disorders
- ❏ Panic Attacks

Relationship Problems
- ❏ Marital, Sexual, Intimacy, Social, Parenting Dysfunction

Self-Abuse
- ❏ Alcohol or Substance Abuse
- ❏ Eating Disorders
- ❏ Self-Injury

II. Process Evaluation*

i. Interpersonal Skills
- ❏ Was aware of patient's nonverbal cues and emotional content
- ❏ Used reflection, checked accuracy of understanding

ii. Information Gathering
- ❏ Asked one question at a time and avoided jargon
- ❏ Used both open-ended and directed questions
- ❏ Clarified and summarized appropriately
- ❏ Ensured that patient understood questions asked
- ❏ Ensured that patient's concerns were addressed and closed interview

*See Global Process Evaluation Criteria (page 10) for a complete evaluation of the interview process.

POST-ENCOUNTER PROBES

Q1. People who have suffered sexual abuse as children may experience sexual-abuse accommodation syndrome. Describe the steps of this syndrome.

i. Secrecy and Silence
ii. Helplessness and Vulnerability
iii. Entrapment and Accommodation
iv. Delayed, Conflicted, and Unconvincing Disclosure
v. Retraction

Q2. To cope with sexual abuse, the child will use immature psychological mechanisms. These mechanisms are thought to be the root cause of adult behaviours seen in sexual-abuse survivors. Name these coping mechanisms.

Self-blame, minimization, denial, fragmentation, dissociation, splitting

Q3. What should physicians do for a patient after disclosure of abuse?

DSM

Document abuse completely and accurately.

Support the abused patient (indicate it is not his/her fault, validate feelings).

Make a safety plan (help person gain access to shelters, legal options, etc.).

Evaluation: Sexually Transmitted Diseases

INSTRUCTIONS FOR CANDIDATE

Svetlana Gorvayewska is 24 years old and is concerned that she may have a sexually transmitted disease (STD). You check her chart and note that three other physicians at your walk-in clinic have seen her this year for dysuria. You cannot find any mention of a Pap test. Perform a directed history.

EVALUATION CRITERIA

I. **History**

  i. **Initial Screen**

- ❏ Currently Sexually Active
- ❏ Orientation (hetero-, homo-, or bisexual)
- ❏ Dating and Past Relationship(s)
- ❏ Number of Past Sexual Partners
- ❏ Current Relationship(s)
- ❏ Number of Current Sexual Partners
- ❏ Sexual Practices (oral, vaginal, anal)
- ❏ Safe Practices and Contraception (frequency of use, types)
- ❏ Awareness of STDs

  ii. **Symptoms of STD—Female**

- ❏ Lower Abdominal and/or Pelvic Pain
- ❏ Cervical Motion Tenderness
- ❏ Adnexal Tenderness
- ❏ Vaginal Discharge
- ❏ Vaginal/Perineal/Perianal Sores, Blisters, or Rash
- ❏ Dysuria
- ❏ Increased Frequency
- ❏ Hematuria

  iii. **Menstrual Symptoms**

- ❏ Age at Menarche
- ❏ Duration of Menses
- ❏ Interval between Periods
- ❏ Amount and Changes in Flow
- ❏ Last Menstrual Period and Recent Changes
- ❏ Dysmenorrhea
- ❏ Infertility

  iv. **Risk Factors for STD and/or Pregnancy**

- ❏ No Use of Barrier Contraception

- ❏ Hx of Previous PID or STDs
- ❏ Multiple Partners
- ❏ New Partner
- ❏ Partner(s) with STD
- ❏ Sex Trade Worker
- ❏ Street Youth

v. Associated Symptoms
- ❏ Fever
- ❏ Chills
- ❏ Night Sweats
- ❏ Rash
- ❏ Swollen Joints
- ❏ Infected Conjunctiva

POST-ENCOUNTER PROBES

Q1. Name five sexually transmitted pathogens and the disease each causes.

Chlamydia trachomatis (chlamydia), *Neisseria gonorrhoeae* (gonorrhea), Herpes simplex virus (herpes), hepatitis B and C (hepatitis), Human Immunodeficiency Virus (HIV/AIDS), *Trepomena pallidum* (syphilis), Human Papilloma Virus (genital warts)

Q2. Describe the signs and symptoms for males and females who have chlamydia and gonorrhea.

	Females	Males
Chlamydia	Dysuria, yellow purulent cervical discharge, joint pain, eye irritation	Dysuria, frequency, urethral discharge, joint pain, eye irritation
Gonorrhea	Dysuria, discharge, abnormal menses, abdom. pain, joint swelling	Dysuria, frequency, purulent urethral discharge, joint swelling

Q3. When taking samples for lab cultures to diagnose an STD such as chlamydia or gonorrhea, what areas are swabbed?

Vaginal/cervical, urethral (male), rectal, and pharyngeal swabs are taken.

Q4. a. What are the physical examinations done for female patients suspected to have an STD?

External genital exam, speculum exam, bimanual exam, and systemic exam (rash, joints) plus swabs

b. What are the physical examinations done for male patients suspected to have an STD?

External genital exam and systemic exam (rash, joints) plus swabs

Q5. What factors may lead you to suspect that an anaerobic infection is the cause of PID in a female patient?

Disease is moderate to severe, prolonged, subacute or chronic; patient is >35 years old, prior PID, IUD is in place, recent gynecological procedure, bacterial vaginosis.

Q6. Teenagers who are at risk for STDs are also at risk for pregnancy. Name three risks of newborns born to teenage mothers.

i.   Failure to thrive
ii. Behavioural problems
iii. Physical abuse

Q7. What are the possible complications of sexually transmitted diseases in females?

Acute salpingitis, PID, infertility, ectopic pregnancies, arthritis, conjunctivitis, urethritis, Fitz-Hugh–Curtis syndrome (chlamydial infection of the liver capsule)

Q8. a. What are the ocular manifestations of Chlamydia trachoma infection?

Keratoconjunctivitis, papillae and follicles on superior palpebral conjunctiva, conjunctival scarring, entropion, corneal abrasions and ulcerations, corneal pannus and blindness

b. How would you treat this infection?

Systemic tetracycline, urgent ophthalmology consultation, and subsequent follow-up

Evaluation: History for Urinary Tract Infection

INSTRUCTIONS FOR CANDIDATE

Martin Nystar is a 16-month-old boy. His mother has noticed that he cries when wetting his diaper, and his urine has a foul smell. Perform a directed history.

EVALUATION CRITERIA

I. **History**

i. **General**
- ❏ Duration of Symptoms
- ❏ Fever/Night Sweats
- ❏ Increased Frequency/Dysuria (number of wet diapers/day)
- ❏ Blood in Diaper
- ❏ Vomiting
- ❏ Diarrhea
- ❏ Feeding Difficulty, Drinking Well
- ❏ Weight Loss

ii. **Risk Factors**
- ❏ Neurogenic Bladder
- ❏ Previously Diagnosed UTI
- ❏ GU Tract Abnormalities (vesicular reflux, single kidney)
- ❏ Diabetes
- ❏ Toilet Training
- ❏ Poor Hygiene
- ❏ Uncircumcised
- ❏ Immunocompromised

iii. **Past Medical History and Family History**
- ❏ Previous UTI
- ❏ Past Urologic Investigations, Surgeries
- ❏ Family Hx of UTI, GU Tract Abnormalities
- ❏ Medications
- ❏ Allergies
- ❏ Immunizations
- ❏ Other Medical Conditions

POST-ENCOUNTER PROBES

Q1. Identify five bacterial agents that cause UTIs in children.

Escherichia coli, Proteus, Streptococcus faecalis, Klebsiella, Pseudomonas, Staphylococcus epidermidis

Q2. What is the differential diagnosis for pyuria?

- Bacterial UTI
- Fever
- Dehydration
- Mycoplasma
- Appendicitis
- Nephritic Syndrome

Q3. What are the grades of vesicoureteral reflux?

Grade 1 — only in ureter

Grade 2 — ureter, pelvis, calyces, no dilatation, normal calyceal fornices

Grade 3 — mild or moderate dilatation and/or tortuosity of ureter, mild or moderate dilatation of the pelvis but no or slight blunting of the fornices

Grade 4 — moderate dilatation and/or tortuosity of the ureter, mild dilatation of renal pelvis and calyces; incomplete obliteration of sharp angle of fornices, but maintenance of papillary impressions in majority of calyces

Grade 5 — gross dilatation and tortuosity of ureter; gross dilatation of renal and pelvis and calyces; papillary impressions no longer visible in majority of calyces

Evaluation: History for Well Baby

INSTRUCTIONS FOR CANDIDATE

Mrs. Holvec is a first-time mother who has brought her daughter, Amy, for her first visit to the doctor. Amy was delivered vaginally at 40 weeks. Perform a directed history.

EVALUATION CRITERIA

I. **History**

    i. **Obstetrical**
- ❑ Gravida, Parity, Spontaneous Abortion, Therapeutic Abortion
- ❑ Duration of Pregnancy
- ❑ Type of Delivery
- ❑ Weight at Birth and Subsequent Weight Gain
- ❑ Neonate Complications and APGAR Score

    ii. **Maternal Health During Pregnancy and Delivery**
- ❑ Gestational Diabetes
- ❑ Hypertension/Hypotension
- ❑ Anemia
- ❑ Number of Ultrasounds
- ❑ Infection/Group B Streptococcus Status
- ❑ EtOH, Drugs (OTC, Rx, and illegal), Tobacco

    iii. **Prenatal Care**
- ❑ Obstetrician, Family Doctor, or Midwife
- ❑ Ultrasound
- ❑ MSS, CVS, and Amniocentesis.

    iv. **Feeding History**
- ❑ Method of Feeding
- ❑ Type of Formula (if not breast fed)
- ❑ Meds Taken by Mother (if breast fed)
- ❑ Difficulty with Feeding; Colic

    v. **Sleep History**
- ❑ Current Sleep Pattern
- ❑ Day Naps
- ❑ Sleep Problems

    vi. **Developmental History**
- ❑ Gross Motor (head control, rolling over, sitting and crawling)
- ❑ Fine Motor (pulls at clothes, reaches, grasps)

- ❑ Speech/Language (coos; responds to voice, babble, and single words)
- ❑ Adaptive/Social (social smile, laugh, stranger anxiety, games)

vii. Past Medical History
- ❑ Congenital Disorders
- ❑ Hospitalizations/Operations
- ❑ Medications
- ❑ Immunizations

viii. Social and Family History
- ❑ Information for Genogram
- ❑ Age of Parents
- ❑ Occupation(s) of Parents/Financial Stability
- ❑ Support Network
- ❑ Significant Family Medical History

POST-ENCOUNTER PROBES

Q1. a. What are the categories measured in developmental milestones?

Gross motor, fine motor, speech/language, and adaptive/social skills

b. For each of the following developmental milestones, provide the age at which they are reached.

Milestone	Age
Walks with support	12 months
Follows simple commands	18 months
Knows 4 colours	5 years
Plays games	9 months
Transfers across midline	8 months
No head lag	4 months

Q2. Name all the vaccinations that children of age 7 should have received if they are "up to date."

Diphtheria, pertussis, tetanus, polio, *H. influenzae,* measles, mumps, and rubella

Q3. a. Define failure to thrive (FTT) as it pertains to a developing child.

FTT is defined as a child weighing less than that of the 3rd percentile, or when the child is less than 80% weight for its height and age.

b. Provide four reasons why FTT may occur.

i.   Inadequate caloric intake is the main underlying factor, which can be caused by reduced intake (swallowing problems, chronic diseases).
ii. Inadequate absorption (celiac disease, CF)
iii. Inappropriate utilization of nutrients (renal loss, inborn errors of metabolism)
iv. Increased requirements (cardiac disease, malignancies, SLE)
v.   Decreased growth potential (fetal alcohol syndrome)

Q4. a. Name three primitive reflexes tested in the neurological exam of a baby.

Palmar grasp, rooting, trunk incurvation, placing response, vertical suspension

b. Which reflex can be pathological at 6 months of age?

Moro reflex

c. What is the Babinski response in newborns and infants?

Toes are upgoing in the normal response.

Q5. What are the measures found in the Apgar score?

Use the acronym How Ready Is The Child?
H — heart rate
R — respiration rate
I — irritability
T — tone/muscle
C — colour

Part III

Scenarios for Directed Histories and Physical Examinations

Evaluation: History and Physical Examination for Acute Abdomen

INSTRUCTIONS FOR CANDIDATE

You are a family physician working in a walk-in clinic. Your next patient, Ms. Watson, comes in complaining of abdominal pain that has been getting progressively worse for the last two days. Perform a directed history and physical examination.

EVALUATION CRITERIA

I. **History**

   i. **Abdominal Pain**

- ❏ Location (localized, diffuse, radiating, referred)
- ❏ Timing (duration, onset, course)
- ❏ Character (quality, quantity)
- ❏ Severity
- ❏ Palliating/Provoking Factors

   ii. **Associated Symptoms**

- ❏ Chills
- ❏ Weight Loss
- ❏ Jaundice
- ❏ Yellow Skin/Sclera
- ❏ Pruritus
- ❏ Pale Stools

   Gastrointestinal

- ❏ Anorexia
- ❏ Nausea
- ❏ Vomiting
- ❏ Diarrhea
- ❏ Constipation
- ❏ Melena
- ❏ Hematochezia
- ❏ Hematemesis
- ❏ Food Intolerance
- ❏ Food Poisoning
- ❏ Travel History

   Changes in Bowel Movements

- ❏ Acute or Chronic Changes
- ❏ Change in Frequency

- [ ] Tenesmus
- [ ] Association with Food
- [ ] Character of Stool

Changes in Bladder Habits
- [ ] Dysuria
- [ ] Changes in Colour of Urine
- [ ] Hematuria
- [ ] Changes in Frequency

Gynecological
- [ ] First Day of Last Menstrual Period
- [ ] Vaginal Discharge
- [ ] Previous STDs
- [ ] IUD Use

Drugs
- [ ] Alcohol
- [ ] NSAIDs
- [ ] Steroids
- [ ] Ulcer Medications

II. Physical Examination

i. General Observations
- [ ] Patient's Positions
- [ ] Level of Distress

ii. Inspection of Skin
- [ ] Colour
- [ ] Scleral Icterus
- [ ] Spider Angiomas

iii. Inspection of Abdomen
- [ ] Contour
- [ ] Symmetry
- [ ] Striae
- [ ] Surgical Scars
- [ ] Visible Peristalsis
- [ ] Umbilical Hernias
- [ ] Cullen's Sign*
- [ ] Grey–Turner's Sign**
- [ ] Angiopathies
- [ ] Caput Medusae

iv. Auscultation
- [ ] Bowel Sounds (normal vs absent)
- [ ] Bruits (renal, aortic, hepatic, com. iliac bifurcation)

v. Percussion
- ❏ Describe Note (tympanic vs dull)
- ❏ Tenderness (often a good substitute for rebound tenderness)
- ❏ Castell's Point or Traub's Space
- ❏ Assesses Shifting Dullness

vi. Palpation
- ❏ Light and Deep Palpation
- ❏ Rebound Pain (Blumberg's sign)
- ❏ Pain on Palpation
- ❏ McBurney's Point Tenderness***
- ❏ Rovsing's Sign****
- ❏ Courvoisier's Sign‡
- ❏ Cough Tenderness
- ❏ Shake Tenderness‡‡
- ❏ Masses

vii. Specific Signs
- ❏ Murphy's Sign‡‡‡
- ❏ Iliopsoas Sign¥
- ❏ Obturator Sign¥¥

*	Cullen's sign: Purple-blue discoloration around umbilicus (peritoneal hemorrhage)
**	Grey–Turner's Sign: Flank discoloration (retroperitoneal hemorrhage)
***	McBurney's point tenderness: One-third from anterior superior iliac spine to umbilicus; if tender, indicates local peritoneal irritation (appendicitis)
****	Rovsing's sign: Palpation pressure to left abdomen causes RLQ McBurney's point tenderness (appendicitis)
‡	Courvoisier's sign: Palpable, nontender gall bladder with jaundice (pancreatic or biliary malignancy)
‡‡	Shake tenderness: Peritoneal irritation, or bump side of bed in suspected malingerers
‡‡‡	Murphy's sign: Inspiratory arrest on deep palpation of RUQ (cholecystitis)
¥	Iliopsoas sign: Flexion of hip against resistance or passive hyperextension of hip causes pain (retrocecal appendix)
¥¥	Obturator sign: Flexion, then external or internal rotation, about the right hip causes pain (pelvic appendicitis)

POST-ENCOUNTER PROBES

Q1. *Give five causes of RUQ pain.*
- Peptic Ulcer
- Pancreatitis
- Hepatitis
- Cholecystitis
- Renal Colic
- Pneumonia/Pleurisy
- Empyema/Pericarditis
- MI

Q2. Name four "red flag" situations that indicate surgery is necessary in the acute abdomen.

- Progressive distention
- Tender mass with fever and hypotension (abscess)
- Septicemia and abdominal findings
- Suspected bowel ischemia (acidosis, fever, and tachycardia)
- Deterioration on conservative treatment

Q3. Percussion and shake tenderness are a sign of what condition?

Peritonitis

Q4. Pain from injury to the viscera in the abdomen often presents as referred pain. In the following pathologies, where is the pain referred?

Biliary Colic — to right shoulder or scapula
Renal Colic — to groin
Appendicitis — epigastric to RLQ
Pancreatitis — to the back
Perforated Ulcer — to RLQ (right paracolic gutter)
Ruptured Aortic Aneurysm — back or flank

Q5. a. Identify the location of McBurney's point on the patient being examined.

One-third of the distance from the anterior superior iliac spine to the umbilicus

b. What is its significance?

Tenderness at this point is a strong indicator that the acute abdomen is caused by appendicitis.

Q6. A young, sexually active female whose period is 3 weeks late presents to your ER with acute abdominal pain. Give three conditions that would be high on your differential diagnosis.

- Ectopic pregnancy
- PID
- Ovarian cyst
- Ovarian torsion

Evaluation: History and Physical Examination for Alcoholism

INSTRUCTIONS FOR CANDIDATE

You are a family doctor working in a rural town. In your previous visit with Mrs. J. Daniels, you determine she has a significant history of alcohol consumption. Perform a directed history and physical examination.

EVALUATION CRITERIA

I. History

i. CAGE Questionnaire

- ❏ Have you ever felt the need to Cut down on your drinking?
- ❏ Have you ever felt Annoyed by criticism of your drinking?
- ❏ Have you ever had Guilty feelings about drinking?
- ❏ Have you ever had an Eye opener (a drink first thing in the morning)?

ii. Assess Drinking Profile

- ❏ What is the setting (time, place, occasion)?
- ❏ Drinks with partners or alone?
- ❏ Ever drink to get high?
- ❏ Pressures to drink?
- ❏ Looks forward to next drink?
- ❏ Unplanned use of alcohol?
- ❏ Protects alcohol supply?
- ❏ Continues to consume greater volumes of alcohol for same effects?
- ❏ Previous attempts to stop drinking?
- ❏ Current or previous symptoms of withdrawal?

iii. Medical Consequences
Physical

- ❏ Fatigue
- ❏ Seizures
- ❏ Blackouts
- ❏ Sleep Disturbance
- ❏ Hypertension
- ❏ Cardiomyopathy
- ❏ Gastritis
- ❏ Peptic Ulcers
- ❏ Gastroesophageal Reflux
- ❏ Pancreatitis

- ❏ Hepatitis
- ❏ Peripheral Neuropathy

Mental
- ❏ Depression
- ❏ Attempted Suicide
- ❏ Family Hx of Alcoholism
- ❏ Other Substance Abuse

iv. Social Consequences
- ❏ Occupation
- ❏ Family
- ❏ Leisure
- ❏ Financial Problems
- ❏ Legal Problems
- ❏ Accidents and Fights
- ❏ Driving Intoxicated

II. Physical Examination
i. Hand
- ❏ Clubbing
- ❏ Palmar Erythema
- ❏ Dupuytren's Contracture
- ❏ Asterixis

ii. Arms
- ❏ Bruising
- ❏ Muscle Atrophy
- ❏ Spider Nevi

iii. Head and Neck
- ❏ Icterus of Sclera
- ❏ Paleness of Conjunctiva
- ❏ Temporal Wasting
- ❏ Parotid Enlargement

iv. Chest
- ❏ Gynecomastia
- ❏ Spider Nevi

v. Abdomen
- ❏ Spider Nevi
- ❏ Caput Medusae
- ❏ Bruising
- ❏ Umbilical Hernia
- ❏ Ascites and Bulging Flanks (flank dullness, shifting dullness or fluid wave)
- ❏ Hepatomegaly (palpates liver edge, percusses liver span)
- ❏ Splenomegaly

III. Process Evaluation*

i. Interpersonal Skills

❑ Was aware of patient's nonverbal cues and emotional content
❑ Used reflection, checked accuracy of understanding

ii. Information Gathering

❑ Asked one question at a time and avoided jargon
❑ Used both open-ended and directed questions
❑ Clarified and summarized appropriately
❑ Ensured that patient understood questions asked
❑ Ensured that patient's concerns were addressed and closed interview

*See Global Process Evaluation Criteria (page 10) for a complete evaluation of the interview process.

POST-ENCOUNTER PROBE

Q1. Identify some alcohol-related medical problems.

GI — esophagitis, gastritis, hepatitis, fatty liver, liver cirrhosis, pancreatitis, peptic ulcers, esophageal or rectal varices, oral and esophageal cancers, and malabsorption

Cardiac — alcoholic cardiomyopathy, arrhythmias

Neurologic — Wernicke's syndrome, Korsakoff's syndrome, cerebellar degeneration

Hematologic — iron or folate anemia, thrombocytopenia, coagulopathies

Endocrine — impotence, hyperlipidemia

Immunologic — immune system impairment

Electrolytes — low calcium, magnesium, or phosphate; ketosis

Q2. What other laboratory markers can be affected by chronic use of alcohol?

Increased MCV, elevated AST>ALT (1.5x), thrombocytopenia

Q3. a. Describe three signs and symptoms of alcohol withdrawal.

Signs and symptoms include autonomic hyperactivity (tachycardia, pyrexia, sweating, tremor, irritability), depressed mood, nausea, vomiting, insomnia, anxiety, seizures, delirium tremens hallucinations (usually visual, but auditory and tactile are possible).

b. When would you expect the onset of these to occur?

Signs and symptoms of alcohol withdrawal occur within 12 to 48 hours after cessation of drinking, but delirium tremens usually occurs within 2 to 10 days.

Q4. Problems with alcohol exist on a continuum. Describe the continuum.

At-Risk Drinking — drinking more than the recommended levels of alcohol (no more than 2 standard drinks per day to a maximum of 9 standard drinks a week for females and 14 standard drinks for males), but no apparent physical or social problems related to alcohol.

Problem Drinking — same as at-risk drinking but with one or more alcohol-related social or physical problems and no clinical features of dependency.

Alcohol Dependency — a maladaptive pattern of alcohol use leading to clinically significant impairment or distress with 3 or more of the following criteria in the past 12 months:

i.   Tolerance
ii. Use of larger amounts of alcohol for longer periods of time
iii. Presence of withdrawal
iv. Symptoms, excessive am't of time spent in obtaining alcohol
v.   Important activities missed or reduced due to alcohol use
vi. Persistent desire but unsuccessful efforts to cut down alcohol

Q5. What is a standard drink?

A standard drink is 13.6 g of alcohol, which is approximately 12 oz of beer (5% alcohol), 5 oz of wine (12%–17% alcohol), 3 oz of fortified wine, or 1.5 oz (80 proof) of liquor.

Evaluation: History and Physical Examination for Asthma

INSTRUCTIONS FOR CANDIDATE

As a general pediatrician, you are called to the Emergency Room to see Letitia Jones, an 8-year-old female whom you have previously admitted to the pediatric Intensive Care Unit because of shortness of breath. Today, the referring ER physician reports that the child once again has shortness of breath and a wheeze. Perform a directed history and physical examination.

EVALUATION CRITERIA

I. History

   i. **General Information**
- ❏ Duration
- ❏ Course
- ❏ Cardiac Disease
- ❏ Foreign Body Aspiration

   ii. **Triggering Factors**
- ❏ URTI
- ❏ Cold Weather
- ❏ Seasonal Allergies
- ❏ Exercise
- ❏ Smoke (in and out of house)
- ❏ Stress
- ❏ Allergens
- ❏ Cats in Residence
- ❏ Gastroesophageal Reflux

   iii. **Asthma History**
- ❏ Number of Admissions
- ❏ ICU Admissions +/– Intubation
- ❏ Frequency of ER Visits
- ❏ Frequency of Beta Agonist Use
- ❏ Current Asthma Medications and Compliance
- ❏ Steroid Dependence and Last Use
- ❏ Symptoms in Specific Environments (school, work)
- ❏ Cough at Night
- ❏ Exercise Tolerance/Cough with Exercise

   iv. **Medical History/Family History**
- ❏ Allergies

- ❏ Immunizations
- ❏ Other Medical Conditions
- ❏ FHx of Asthma, Eczema, Hay Fever

II. Physical Examination
i. General
- ❏ Ability to Speak (full sentence vs single words)
- ❏ Restlessness
- ❏ Altered Mental Status
- ❏ Fatigue
- ❏ Vital Signs (RR, HR, BP, O_2 saturation)
- ❏ Pulsus Paradoxus
- ❏ Cyanosis

ii. Respiratory
- ❏ Barrel Chest
- ❏ Cough
- ❏ Accessory Muscle Use
- ❏ Air Entry
- ❏ Wheezes and Location
- ❏ Crackles and Location
- ❏ Percussion—Hypertympanic
- ❏ Prolonged Expiration
- ❏ Clubbing

iii. Focus of Infection
- ❏ Rhinorrhea, Coryza
- ❏ Pharynx
- ❏ Tympanic Membrane
- ❏ Cardiovascular Examination
- ❏ Abdominal Examination
- ❏ Skin Examination—Rash

POST-ENCOUNTER PROBE

Q1. List three investigations you would perform and why.

Oxygen Saturation — to determine if patient needs supplemental oxygen

Arterial Blood Gas or **Capillary Blood Gas** — to determine if patient is in impending respiratory failure

CX—if suspicious of pneumothorax, pneumonia, or foreign-body aspiration

Peak Flow — to determine degree of compromise of respiratory function

Q2. Discuss treatment of asthma and the point at which you would escalate treatment.

i. Environmental control and education
ii. Inhaling short-acting beta-2 agonist prn

iii. Adding inhaled steroid if required (beta-2 agonist > 3–4 times per week)
iv. Increasing dose of inhaled steroid if still requiring beta-2 agonist > 3–4 times per week
v. Additional Tx — long-acting beta-2 agonists and/or leukotriene-receptor antagonists
vi. Oral prednisone.

Q3. What is the treatment of an acute asthma exacerbation?

- Supplemental oxygen if needed
- Salbutamol by aerosol mask
- Ipratropium bromide proven beneficial if given with salbutamol for first three aerosol masks
- Oral or intravenous corticosteroids if moderate-to-severe exacerbation
- IV fluids if dehydrated
- Consider admission

Evaluation: History and Physical Examination for Back Pain

INSTRUCTIONS FOR CANDIDATE

Mr. McCallum, one of your regular patients in your family medicine practice, comes to you complaining of increasing low back pain that began 5 days ago. Perform a directed history and physical examination.

EVALUATION CRITERIA

I. **History**

   i. **Pain**
- ❏ Location
- ❏ Onset
- ❏ Duration
- ❏ Association with Trigger Event (e.g., trauma, lifting)
- ❏ Worse in Leg or Back?
- ❏ Quality (shooting or aching, constant vs intermittent)
- ❏ Quantity and Severity of Attacks
- ❏ Changes with Position
- ❏ Pattern (worse with flexion/extension/walking; day/night)
- ❏ Progression (Is the pain getting better or worse?)
- ❏ Alleviating/Aggravating Factors (specific positions, with use, etc.)

   ii. **Associated Symptoms**

     Constitutional Symptoms
- ❏ Fever
- ❏ Fatigue
- ❏ Night Sweats
- ❏ Weight Loss
- ❏ Chills

     Bladder Symptoms
- ❏ Urinary Retention
- ❏ Increased Frequency
- ❏ Overflow Incontinence
- ❏ Hesitancy

     Bowel Symptoms
- ❏ Incontinence
- ❏ Poor Sphincter Control

     Myelopathy
- ❏ Perianal or Saddle Anesthesia

❏   Loss of Sensation in Legs
❏   Leg Weakness
❏   Erectile Dysfunction

iii. Medical History
❏   Back Pain
❏   Malignancy (cancer of the thyroid, kidney, breast, prostate, or lungs)
❏   Vascular Diseases
❏   Seropositive or Seronegative Disease
❏   Immunosuppression
❏   Osteoporosis

iv. Impact on Life
❏   Occupation (sitting or standing all day)
❏   Limitations in Usual Activities
❏   Interference with Sleep/Social Activities/Occupation
❏   How Long Can Patient Sit/Stand/Walk?
❏   How Much Weight Can Patient Lift?

II. Physical Examination
i. Inspection (cervical, thoracic, and lumbar curves)
❏   Symmetry
❏   Edema
❏   Deformity:
❏   Lordosis
❏   Kyphosis
❏   Scoliosis
❏   Differences in Heights of Shoulders and Iliac Crests
❏   Rib Hump
❏   Signs of Inflammation
❏   Signs of Trauma
❏   Scars
❏   Abnormal Gait

ii. Palpation (spinous processes)
❏   Tenderness
❏   Prominence
❏   Alignment
❏   Paravertebral Muscle Tenderness
❏   Tenderness over Spinous Processes

iii. Range of Motion
❏   Forward Flexion (herniation, range of motion)
❏   Extension (facet joint, range of motion)
❏   Lateral Flexion (range of motion)
❏   Rotation (range of motion)
❏   Chest Expansion (difference between inspiration and expiration)

iv. Neurological (Nerve Root) Screen
Motor
- ❏ Squat and Rise (L4)
- ❏ Heel Walking (L5)
- ❏ Walking on Toes (S1)

Sensory
- ❏ Medial Calf (L4)
- ❏ 1st Web Space (L5)
- ❏ Lateral Foot (S1)

Reflex
- ❏ Knee Jerk (L4)
- ❏ Ankle Jerk (S1)

v. Special Tests
- ❏ Straight Leg Raise (Lesague test for L4, 5; S1, 2, 3 nerve roots)
- ❏ Femoral Stretch Test (L2, 3, 4 nerve roots)
- ❏ Hip Screen

vi. Peripheral Vascular System
- ❏ Femoral Pulse
- ❏ Femoral Bruits
- ❏ Distal Pulses

POST-ENCOUNTER PROBES

Q1. Identify two surgical emergencies that can cause lower back symptoms.

Cauda equina syndrome; abdominal aortic aneurysm/rupture

Q2. What are the neurological deficits of cauda equina syndrome?

Saddle anesthesia, decreased anal tone, perianal sensory loss, fecal incontinence, urinary retention, severe or progressive neurological deficit

Q3. a. Name four medical conditions that can cause lower back symptoms.

Neoplastic — primary, metastatic

Inflammatory — seronegative/spondyloarthropathies

Metabolic — osteoporosis with fractures, osteomalacia, Paget's disease

Infectious — osteomyelitis, TB

Visceral — prostatitis, endometriosis, pyelonephritis, pancreatitis

b. Classify low back pain.

Urgent (Red Flag) Spinal Conditions — as mentioned in (a)

Sciatica — back and lower limb symptoms suggestive of lumbosacral nerve root compromise

Other — nonspecific back symptoms

Q4. Name some red flags that may indicate potential serious etiologies of low back pain.

Constitutional symptoms; history of recent bacterial infections, malignancies, trauma, or inflammatory diseases; bowel or bladder dysfunction; saddle anesthesia; IV drug use; chronic disease; neurological deficits; age >50 years

Q5. a. What three special physical techniques can be used to identify sciatica?

Straight leg raise, crossover pain, sitting knee extension

b. When is sciatic pain caused by nerve root compression operable?

Consider surgery when sciatic pain is severe and disabling, lasting >4 weeks, or has rapid progression, and imaging studies confirm an intervertebral disc herniation that accounts for the sciatica.

Q6. How can one distinguish between lumbar spinal stenosis and lumbar disc prolapse?

Spinal stenosis often causes neurogenic claudication. Radiculopathy, paresthesia, and weakness provoked by activity and palliated by sitting, bending over, or lying down characterize neurogenic claudication. Also, special tests for sciatic pain are often negative, with objective neurological findings after exercise.

Q7. Outline five steps of a treatment plan you have for a patient with low back pain.

i.   Use acetaminophen as first line for pain relief. NSAIDs and ASA are also good pain meds but have more side effects. Avoid opiates, especially chronic opiate use.

ii.   Alter activities: bed rest for maximum of 2–4 days if severe limitation due to leg pain.

iii. Avoid lifting, twisting, bending, and prolonged sitting. Education about proper lifting, carrying, etc.

iv.   Change positions frequently; use soft supports for the lumbar spine and a reclining position when sitting.

v.   Avoid debilitation with use of conditioning exercises such as walking, stationary cycling, swimming, and light jogging. Start within first 2 weeks of symptoms and graduate level up to 30 minutes daily. Specific conditioning exercises are not useful in the first 2–3 weeks of injury but play a role in maintaining conditioning and exercise tolerance.

Evaluation: History and Physical Examination for Breast Lump

INSTRUCTIONS FOR CANDIDATE

As an intern doing your internal medicine rotation, you are taking care of Mrs. Pellegrini, a 55-year-old female whom you are treating for congestive heart failure. Today, while you are doing your regular rounds, she tells you that she has felt a lump in her left breast. Perform a directed history and physical examination.

EVALUATION CRITERIA

I. History

i. Breast Lump

❑ Location of Lump (quadrant, distance from nipple, L vs R)
❑ Onset, Timing, Duration for Presence of Lump
❑ Changes with Respect to Menstrual Cycle (size, shape, pain)
❑ Associated Pain
❑ Physical Features:
❑   Shape (round, oval, etc.)
❑   Consistency (soft, firm, hard, cystic, solid, etc.)
❑   Mobility
❑   Delineation (discrete, fixed)
❑   Recent Breast Injury

ii. Associated Signs and Symptoms

❑ Nipple Discharge (amount, colour, smell)
❑ Nipple Retraction
❑ Skin Changes (discoloration, induration, erythema, dimpling)
❑ Breast Size Changes
❑ Auxillary Lumps and Swelling, Arm Swelling
❑ Fever
❑ Weight Loss
❑ Chills

iii. Risk Factors

❑ Family Hx of Breast/Ovarian Cancer
❑ Past Hx of Breast Cancer
❑ Prior Breast Biopsy
❑ Age of Menarche
❑ Age of Menopause
❑ Nulliparity
❑ Parity, Age of 1st Born

❏ Obesity
❏ Excessive Alcohol Intake
❏ Radiation Exposure

iv. Symptoms Associated with Metastasis
❏ Brain (changes in personality, hearing, sight, and/or memory)
❏ Lung (SOB, cough, hemoptysis)
❏ Bone (pain, fractures)

II. Physical Examination
i. Inspection (Breast)
(Done with patient sitting with arms at her sides, raised over her head, pressing on her hips, and leaning forward)
❏ Size
❏ Symmetry
❏ Colour
❏ Visible Masses
❏ Shape Changes (abnormal bulging)
❏ Skin Retraction, Dimpling, or Flattening
❏ Ulceration or Eczema
❏ Erythema
❏ Peau d'Orange
❏ Increased Vascularity

ii. Inspection (Areola and Nipple)
❏ Size
❏ Shape (retracted nipple)
❏ Symmetry (deviated nipple)
❏ Ulceration or Eczema (Paget's disease)
❏ Discharge (serous, bloody, milky, clear, etc.)
❏ Supernumerary Nipples

iii. Palpation (Cervical, Supraclavicular, Infraclavicular, Axillary Nodes)
❏ Location
❏ Size and Shape
❏ Consistency
❏ Mobility

iv. Bilateral Breast Exam
❏ Examines each breast separately
❏ Drapes the breast that is not being examined
❏ Uses pads of the fingers (usually 2nd, 3rd, and 4th fingers)
❏ Palpates at three different levels (light, medium, deep)
❏ Asks patient if she feels any pain on palpation
❏ Uses the vertical strip or radial strip method
❏ Keeps fingers on the breast at all times
❏ Palpates entire breast including periphery, nipple, areola, and tail
❏ Asks patient to express nipple discharge

POST-ENCOUNTER PROBES

Q1. How do you differentiate between a benign and a malignant lump clinically?

Benign — smooth, rubbery (soft), mobile, well-demarcated, tender

Malignant — irregular, poorly defined, less mobile, hard, painless, peau d'orange ± tethering

Q2. What are the signs and symptoms of breast cancer?

- Palpable mass
- Breast swelling and pain
- Skin dimpling, retraction, or ulceration
- Edema (arm or breast)
- Erythema
- Nipple discharge (esp. bloody), retraction, crusting, or ulceration
- Prominent veins
- Palpable axillary/supraclavicular lymph nodes

Q3. What mammographic findings are suggestive of malignancy?

- Microcalcification
- Irregular stellate or spiculated mass
- Architectural distortion
- Increased vascularity
- Interval mammographic changes

Q4. a. What is the staging of breast cancer?

Stage 0 — carcinoma in situ

Stage 1 — tumour <2 cm

Stage 2 — tumour >5 cm without nodes or between 2–5 cm with or without ipsilateral nodes or <2 cm with ipsilateral nodes

Stage 3 — any size with fixed ipsilateral or internal mammary nodes or tumour of any size invading skin or chest wall

Stage 4 — tumour of any size with distant metastasis

b. What is the corresponding management for each stage of breast cancer?

Treatment for:

Stage 0 — includes excision with clear margins and possibly radiation therapy

Stage 1 — includes lumpectomy with axillary node dissection and radiation or total mastectomy with axillary node dissection. Use of adjuvant therapy, including tamoxifen, depends upon presence of estrogen receptors.

Combination chemotherapy, including cyclophosphamide, methotrexate and 5-fluorouracil, is used with estrogen-receptor–negative tumours or in premenopausal women with estrogen-positive tumours and positive lymph nodes.

Stage 2 — same as for stage 1

Stage 3 — operate for local control*

Stage 4 — same as for stage 3

* Tumours >5 cm, those that invade the chest wall or skin, or inflammatory carcinomas are treated with induction chemotherapy.

Evaluation: History and Physical Examination for Chest Pain

INSTRUCTIONS FOR CANDIDATE

Mr. Singh comes rushing into your ER with his 64-year-old wife, who is complaining of sudden onset of severe chest discomfort over the last 30 minutes. Perform a directed history and physical examination.

EVALUATION CRITERIA

I. **History**

i. **Chest Pain**
- ❏ Location (localized, diffuse, radiating, referred)
- ❏ Timing (duration, onset, course)
- ❏ Character (quality, quantity)
- ❏ Severity
- ❏ Palliating/Provoking Factors (amount of activity before onset)

ii. **Associated Symptoms**
- ❏ Fever
- ❏ Edema (ankle, sacral, lungs)
- ❏ Syncope
- ❏ Dyspnea/Orthopnea
- ❏ Cough
- ❏ Hemoptysis
- ❏ Palpitations
- ❏ Nocturia
- ❏ Leg Pain
- ❏ Nausea and Vomiting

iii. **Risk Factors for Atherosclerotic Heart Disease**
- ❏ Smoking
- ❏ Diabetes
- ❏ Hypertension
- ❏ Hyperlipidemia
- ❏ Family History
- ❏ Lifestyle (active vs sedentary)

iv. **Past Medical History**
- ❏ Medications and Allergies
- ❏ Smoking and Alcohol Intake
- ❏ Hospitalizations
- ❏ Cardiac Illnesses (rheumatic heart disease)
- ❏ Cardiac Surgeries

II. Physical Examination

i. General Inspection

❏ Level of Distress
❏ Colour (cyanotic, pale, grey)
❏ Vital Signs (pulse, BP, respiration rate, O_2 sat.)

ii. Inspection

❏ Markings (scars, wounds, pacemakers)
❏ Visible Pulsations

iii. Palpation

❏ PMI (location, size, duration)
❏ Lifts, Heaves, and Thrills

iv. Auscultation

❏ Supine (S1, S2; all 5 areas with bell and diaphragm)
❏ Upright (S1, S2; all 5 areas with bell and diaphragm)
❏ Left Lat. Decubitus (S3, S4 with bell)
❏ Lean Forward (diastolic murmurs with bell at the base of the heart)

POST-ENCOUNTER PROBES

Q1. a. What is syncope?

Syncope is the sudden, transient loss of consciousness with loss of postural tone.

b. What are palpitations?

Sensations of an unduly rapid or irregular heartbeat

c. In what circumstances might normal, healthy people be aware of their heart beating?

Exercise and states of anxiety

Q2. What signs and symptoms would you expect to find if part of the left anterior descending artery was occluded?

The LAD artery usually supplies the left side of the heart, and in left-sided heart failure one would expect to find: dyspnea, orthopnea, basal crackles in the lungs, cough, hemoptysis, fatigue, syncope, systemic hypotension, cool extremities, and peripheral cyanosis.

Q3. What signs and symptoms would you expect to find if part of the right coronary vessel was occluded?

The RCA usually supplies the right side of the heart, and in right-sided heart failure one would expect to find: peripheral edema, hepatic tenderness, hepatomegaly, pulsatile liver, elevated JVP, and positive hepatojugular reflux.

Q4. Provide a differential diagnosis of chest pain.

Cardiovascular — coronary artery disease, angina/MI, aortic aneurysm/ dissection

Pulmonary — pneumothorax, pleurisy, pulmonary embolus, pneumonia

Gastrointestinal — esophagitis, hiatus hernia, peptic ulcer, pancreatitis, cholecystitis

Musculoskeletal — costochondrodynia, muscle spasm, nonspecific chest-wall pain

Other — anxiety, herpes zoster

Q5. Provide six steps of treatment for patients with acute coronary artery disease.

Ensure airway, breathing, and circulation (ABCs); start telemetry; get an EKG; draw blood for cardiac enzymes; gain intravenous access; start drug therapy (including oxygen, ASA, nitroglycerin, morphine, and beta blockers); and reassess the patient.

Evaluation: History and Physical Examination for Congestive Heart Failure

INSTRUCTIONS FOR CANDIDATE

Juan Gonzalez is a 78-year-old man with a significant smoking history and chronic obstructive pulmonary disease. He has survived three myocardial infarctions over the last ten years. He is often seen by physicians at your clinic for respiratory complaints. Today, he has come to see you for worsening shortness of breath and ankle swelling. Perform a directed history and physical examination.

EVALUATION CRITERIA

I. **History**

   i. **Dyspnea**
- ❏ Timing (duration, onset, course)
- ❏ Character (severity at rest; with exertion)
- ❏ Orthopnea (no. pillows used to sleep)
- ❏ Paroxysmal Nocturnal Dyspnea
- ❏ Baseline Level of Functioning/Exercise Tolerance

   ii. **Associated Symptoms**
- ❏ Fatigue
- ❏ Fever
- ❏ Diaphoresis
- ❏ Presyncope/Syncope
- ❏ Dyspnea/Orthopnea
- ❏ Cough
- ❏ Hemoptysis
- ❏ Palpitations
- ❏ Nocturia
- ❏ Nausea
- ❏ Edema (ankle, sacral, lungs)
- ❏ Weight Gain

   iii. **Precipitants of CHF**
- ❏ Hypertension
- ❏ Endocarditis
- ❏ Environment (heat/humidity)
- ❏ Anemia
- ❏ Rheumatic Heart Disease or Valve Disease
- ❏ Thyrotoxicosis
- ❏ Pregnancy

- ❏ Failure with Medication Compliance
- ❏ Arrhythmia
- ❏ Infection/Ischemia/Infarction
- ❏ Lung Disease (pulmonary embolism, COPD, pneumonia)
- ❏ Endocrinopathy (hyperthyroidism, pheochromocytoma, Conn's syndrome)
- ❏ Dietary Noncompliance (high salt, fluid, alcohol)

II. Physical Examination

i. General Inspection
- ❏ Respiratory Distress
- ❏ Anxiety

ii. Vital Signs
- ❏ Tachycardia
- ❏ Tachypnea
- ❏ Hyper-/Hypotension
- ❏ Elevated JVP (abdominal jugular reflux present)

iii. Chest
- ❏ Percussion Note Dullness (pleural effusion)
- ❏ Auscultation (crackles, rhonchi)

iv. Heart
- ❏ Palpation (displacement of apex)
- ❏ Auscultation (irregular rhythm, S3)

v. Abdomen
- ❏ Inspection (ascites)
- ❏ Palpation (hepatomegaly and liver tenderness)

vi. Extremities
- ❏ Inspection (pedal/sacral edema, jaundice, muscle wasting)
- ❏ Palpation (pedal/sacral edema)

POST-ENCOUNTER PROBES

Q1. Describe the New York scale of classifying congestive heart failure.

Class I — Exercise/Exertion Exacerbates Symptoms

Class II — Usual Level of ADLs Exacerbate Symptoms

Class III — Minimal ADLs Exacerbate Symptoms (asymptomatic at rest)

Class IV — Symptomatic at Rest

Q2. List several conditions that may provoke congestive heart failure.

CAD, MI, hypertension, valvular disease (aortic/mitral), cardiomyopathy, myocarditis, brady-/tachyarrhythmias, conditions of increased output (anemia, hyperthyroidism), renal failure, nephrotic syndrome

Q3. What basic investigations would you order to work up a patient whom you suspect has congestive heart failure?

Routine blood work, including an assessment of renal and hepatic function, EKG, CXR, and assessment of ventricular size and function by echocardiogram or nuclear medicine studies

Q4. Identify the basic principles in managing congestive heart failure.

- Symptomatic measures (oxygen and bed rest)
- Controlling salt and fluid balance (decreasing salt and fluids, using diuretics)
- Vasodilation (arteriodilation—afterload reduction; venodilation—preload reduction)
- Inotropic medications (digoxin, sympathomimetics)
- Beta-blockers, calcium channel blockers, antiarrhythmics

Q5. You are caring for a patient who has had a first-time exacerbation of congestive heart failure with mild dyspnea at rest 5 days ago. Suggest seven nonpharmacologic and/or pharmacologic treatment options you would ensure for this patient before discharging him or her.

i. Aggressive risk factor management (Optimize control of diabetes mellitus, hyperlipidemia, smoking cessation, etc.)
ii. Lifestyle modifications (Decrease salt and alcohol in diet, reduce weight, advise regarding exercise.)
iii. Salt and fluid monitoring
iv. Tailored diuretic use
v. Starting ACE inhibitors
vi. Starting ß-blocker.
vii. Starting spironolactone
viii. Starting digoxin
ix. Arranging appropriate multidisciplinary follow-up and education (Patient to see dietitian, physiotherapist, occupational therapist, nurse practitioners, pharmacists, family doctor, cardiologist, other specialists as needed, support groups)

Q6. What are your exercise recommendations for a person with congestive heart failure and a stable NYHA functional class I, II, or III?

- Make sure everyone with stable NYHA functional class I, II, or III exercises regularly.
- Arrange a cardiologic stress test before beginning an exercise program.
- Individualize the exercise program for each patient. Sicker patients should start at lower-intensity exercises for shorter sessions.
- Make both resistance training and aerobic training equally important parts of any fitness regime.

Evaluation: History and Physical Examination for Cough

INSTRUCTIONS FOR CANDIDATE

As a family physician, you are about to see a new patient by the name of Joanne Warner. Your nurse tells you that she is 32 years old and was the unfortunate victim of a car accident ten years ago which left her paraplegic. Otherwise, she was in good health until four days ago, when she developed a productive cough and mild dyspnea. Perform a directed history and physical examination.

EVALUATION CRITERIA

I. **History**

   i. **Cough**
- [ ] Duration
- [ ] Onset
- [ ] Frequency
- [ ] Change over Time
- [ ] Quality (dry vs productive)
- [ ] Sputum Characteristics (hemoptysis, volume)
- [ ] Palliating/Provoking Factors

   ii. **Associated Symptoms**
- [ ] Constitutional Symptoms (fever, chills, weight loss)
- [ ] Chest Pain
- [ ] Characteristics of Pain (pleuritic vs visceral, duration, onset)
- [ ] Palliating and Provoking Factors for Pain
- [ ] Limitations and Changes in Baseline Functioning
- [ ] Dyspnea and Orthopnea

   iii. **Risk Factors**
- [ ] Smoking (pack-year Hx)
- [ ] Occupation Hx (smoke, chemical, or irritant exposures)
- [ ] Family Hx of Lung Cancer or Other Cancers
- [ ] Exposure to Person(s) with Lung Infections
- [ ] TB Status
- [ ] Recent Travel Hx

   iv. **Medical History**
- [ ] Medications and Allergies
- [ ] Chronic Lung Disease (asthma, COPD, cystic fibrosis)
- [ ] Chronic Heart Disease (CHF, MI, arrhythmias)

- ☐   Past Hospitalizations and Surgeries
- ☐   Other Chronic Illnesses

II.   Physical Examination
i.   Inspection
- ☐   Facial Expression
- ☐   Acute Distress (stridor/wheeze)
- ☐   Cyanosis
- ☐   Nasal Flaring/Pursed Lip Breathing
- ☐   Accessory Muscle Use
- ☐   Paradoxical Respiration
- ☐   Respiration Rate and Pattern
- ☐   Hands (cigarette stains)

Palpation
- ☐   Palpation for Tenderness
- ☐   Chest Excursion
- ☐   Tactile Fremitus

Percussion
- ☐   All Lung Fields plus Supraclavicular Fossa
- ☐   Description of Percussion Note
- ☐   Diaphragmatic Excursion

Auscultation
- ☐   Description of Sounds in all Fields (intensity, pitch, adventitious)
- ☐   Special Manoeuvres for Consolidation:
- ☐   Bronchophony
- ☐   Pectorioloquy
- ☐   Egophony

POST-ENCOUNTER PROBE

Q1. a. What are you looking for when you are examining accessory muscles?

Looking for motion in scalene muscles, sternocleidomastoid muscles, neck-strap muscles, intercostal muscles, and abdominal motion when person inspires

b. What accessory muscle group is the earliest muscle recruited in respiration?

Scalene muscles

c. What might one observe with this type of breathing at the intercostal spaces and supraclavicular fossa?

Indrawing

d. What is paradoxical respiration?

The abdomen draws inward on inspiration when it normally should move outward due to diaphragm descent.

Q2. Provide a differential diagnosis for:

a. cough

Airway Irritants — inhaled smoke, dusts, fumes, aspiration of gastric contents, oral and nasal secretions, foreign body

Airway Disease —acute/chronic bronchitis, bronchiectasis, neoplasm, asthma, COPD

Parenchyma Disease — pneumonia, lung abscess, interstitial lung disease

Cardiac — mitral valve stenosis, congestive heart failure

Drug- or Toxin-Induced — ACE inhibitors, smoking

b. dyspnea

Airway Disease — upper/lower airway obstruction (anaphylaxis, foreign body), asthma, COPD, mucus plugging

Parenchymal — pneumonia, pneumoconiosis, adult respiratory distress

Pleural Disease — pneumothorax, pleural effusion

Pulmonary Vascular Occlusion — pulmonary embolus (clot, fat, amniotic), pulmonary hypertension, pulmonary vasculitis

Diseases of the Respiratory Pump — kyphoscoliosis, flail chest, c-spine injuries, neuromuscular diseases (myasthenia gravis, Guillain-Barre syndrome, polio)

Cardiac — CHF, ischemia of heart, arrhythmias, mitral valve stenosis

Anxiety

Metabolic — anemia

Q3. Name the common bacteria that cause pneumonia.

Typical Bacteria— *S. pneumoniae, S. pyogenes, H. influenzae, M. catarrhalis*

Atypical Bacteria— *Chlamydia pneumoniae, Mycoplasma, Legionella, C. burnettii*

Q4. Give three pieces of
a. historical information,
b. physical findings, and
c. laboratory criteria that you would find useful in determining admission for a patient that you suspect has a pneumonia.

a.   Age of patient, history of co-morbid illnesses (neoplasm, liver, CHF, CVA, renal disease)

b.   Altered mental status, respiration rate >30/min, systolic BP <90, temperature <36°C or >40°C, tachycardia >125 bpm

c.   Blood pH <7.35, BUN >10.7 mmol/L, Na <130 mmol/L, glucose >13.9 mmol/L, hematocrit <30%, PO_2 <90%, pleural effusion

Evaluation: History and Physical Examination for Craniofacial Trauma

INSTRUCTIONS FOR CANDIDATE

Jesus Cordova was driving in his minivan (without wearing his seatbelt) when he suddenly had to slam on his brakes to avoid hitting a deer. He is brought to the hospital where you, the ER resident, are asked to assess him. He complains of seeing double when looking left and of being unable to close his jaw. Perform a directed history and physical examination.

EVALUATION CRITERIA

I. **History**
- ❏ History of Events Leading to Facial Trauma
- ❏ History of Previous Facial Trauma
- ❏ Previous and Current Occular Findings (visual acuity and diplopia)
- ❏ Facial Paresthesia/Paralysis
- ❏ Malocclusion

   Medical History
- ❏ Medications and Allergies
- ❏ Medical Conditions and Past Surgeries
- ❏ Last Meal

II. **Physical Examination**
   i. **Airway/Breathing/Circulation**
   ii. **C-Spine Assessment**
   iii. **General Inspection**
- ❏ Deformity/Symmetry
- ❏ Edema
- ❏ Lacerations
- ❏ Hematomas
- ❏ Bleeding (hemotympanum/epistaxis)
- ❏ Exophthalmos/Enophthalmos
- ❏ Basal Skull Fracture (raccoon eyes, Battle's sign, CSF otorrhea)

   iv. **Palpation**
- ❏ Tenderness, Step Deformities, Crepitus in:
- ❏   Supraorbital and Infraorbital Rim
- ❏   Maxilla and Malar Region
- ❏   Mandible

❏   Palate Stability
❏   Carotid Arteries
❏   v. **Cranial Nerve Screens (see Physical Examination of Cranial Nerves on page 167)**

POST-ENCOUNTER PROBES

Q1. Describe the potential ocular emergencies involved in facial trauma.

Superior Orbital Fissure Syndrome — involves cranial nerves III–VI and superior ophthalmic vein; needs immediate surgical decompression to prevent permanent nerve damage

Orbital Apex Syndrome — same as above scenario, but the optic nerve is also involved

Q2. What are serious syndromes that must be ruled out in craniofacial trauma?

Diplopia, enophthalmos, blindness, CSF leakage, sinusitis, cranial nerve palsies, poor cosmesis, functional impairments

Evaluation: History and Physical Examination for Dementia

INSTRUCTIONS FOR CANDIDATE

You are a family doctor for a local retirement home. A concerned son of one of your patients has asked you to assess his father, Giovanni D'Amico, who is 78 years old. The son is concerned about increasing lapses in his father's memory. Perform a directed history and physical examination.

EVALUATION CRITERIA

I. **History**

   i. **Initial Screen**
- ❏ Assesses Hearing/Vision
- ❏ Assesses Orientation (person, place, time)
- ❏ Elicits Chief Complaint

   ii. **Description of Symptoms**
- ❏ Onset, Duration, and Course of Current Complaint(s)
- ❏ Palliating/Provoking Factors
- ❏ Limitations in Functioning (ADLs, IADLs)

   iii. **Depression Symptoms**
- ❏ Assesses Depression Symptoms (low mood, anhedonia, sleep disturbance, etc.)
- ❏ Assesses Suicidality and Homicidality

   iv. **Anxiety Symptoms**
- ❏ Anxiety Symptoms (phobias, obsessions, compulsions, etc.)

   v. **Perception Disturbances**
- ❏ Psychotic Symptoms (hallucinations, delusions, ideas of reference, etc.)

   vi. **Personality and Behavioural Disturbances**
- ❏ Changes in Personality
- ❏ Behavioural Abnormalities (apathy, agitation, odd behaviours, etc.)

   vii. **Past and Family Medical History**
- ❏ Hx of Alcohol/Drug Abuse
- ❏ Medications and Hx of Adverse Drug Reactions
- ❏ Hx of Psychiatric Illness
- ❏ Hx of Other Metabolic or Systemic Illness(es)

viii. Collateral History from Family Member
- ❏ Elicits Concerns
- ❏ Confirms History
- ❏ Inquires about Safety, Home Fire Risks, Driving, Wandering

II. Physical Examination
i. Inspection (Candidates should comment on)
- ❏ Dress and Grooming
- ❏ Speech
- ❏ Attitude and Behaviour in Office

ii. Folstein Mini-Mental Status Exam
- ❏ Orientation (place, time: 5 pt for each)
- ❏ Registration (name 3 objects: 1 pt for each)
- ❏ Attention and Concentration (serial 7's, world, months: 5 pt total)
- ❏ Recall (recall 3 objects: 1 pt for each)
- ❏ Language
- ❏ (identify 2 objects pointed to: 2 pt total).
- ❏ (ask no ifs, ands, or buts: 1 pt total)
- ❏ (perform 3-stage command: 3 pt total)
- ❏ (read and obey written command: 1 pt total)
- ❏ (write a sentence: 1 pt total)
- ❏ (draw intersecting pentagons: 1 pt total)
- ❏ Provide Patient's Score and Its Interpretation

iii. Additional Cognitive Tests
- ❏ Perseveration (ask patient to copy a series of loops)
- ❏ Construction Ability (draw hands of clock for diff. times)
- ❏ Concrete Thinking (compare word similarities)
- ❏ Abstract Thinking (describe meaning of proverb)

III. Process Evaluation*
i. Interpersonal Skills
- ❏ Was aware of patient's nonverbal cues and emotional content
- ❏ Used reflection, checked accuracy of understanding

ii. Information Gathering
- ❏ Asked one question at a time and avoided jargon
- ❏ Used both open-ended and directed questions
- ❏ Clarified and summarized appropriately
- ❏ Ensured that patient understood questions asked
- ❏ Ensured that patient's concerns were addressed and closed interview

*See Global Process Evaluation Criteria (page 10) for a complete evaluation of the interview process.

POST-ENCOUNTER PROBES

Q1. a. What is an abnormal Folstein Mini-Mental Status score?

This exam is a screening test only and has false positives. This is the reason that an assessment of functioning is also needed to confirm a diagnosis of dementia. A score of less than 24 indicates impaired mental functioning.

b. Give three reasons other than dementia that could also explain a low score.

Amotivation, poor concentration, poor education, difficulties understanding the examiner's language, sensory impairments (e.g., decreased visual acuity, hearing impairment, etc.)

c. Identify four activities of daily living (ADLs) and four instrumental activities of daily living (IADLs).

ADLs—Dressing, Eating, Ambulation, Toileting and Transfers, Hygiene (**DEATH**)

IADLs—Shopping, Housework, Accounting (banking), Food preparation, Transportation (**SHAFT**)

Q2. How can one differentiate between delirium and dementia?

	Delirium	**Dementia**
Onset:	Rapid	Progressive
Course:	Fluctuates over time	Constant or may slowly worsen
Orientation:	Disoriented to time and place	Disoriented to time and place usually only in late stages
Psychosis:	More likely present	Less likely present
Other:	Perceptual disturbances, sleep–wake cycles disturbed, incr. or decr. psychomotor activity	Loss of judgment, changes in personality present
Reversible:	Often	Very rarely

Q3. What is the differential diagnosis for dementia?

D—drugs (alcohol, barbiturates, bromides)

E—emotion (depression, schizophrenia)

M—metabolic (Wernicke-Korsakoff syndrome, B_{12}/folate deficiency, hyper/hypothyroid)

E—eye and ear (severe visual and auditory impairment)

N—neurodegenerative (Huntington's, Parkinson's, Alzheimer's disease)

T—trauma (head injury, dementia pugilistica), tumour (subfrontal meningioma)

I—infection (HIV, syphilis, viral encephalitis, Creutzfeld–Jacob disease)

A—arteriosclerotic and vascular (multi-infarct dementia, vasculitis, cerebral hemorrhage)

Q4. What is the single best means to diagnose dementia in a patient?

A thorough history and clinical mental status examination, which may need to be repeated at intervals of 3 to 6 months to confirm the progressive nature of dementia

Q5. a. What are the essential laboratory investigations you would order to confirm your diagnosis of dementia?

CBC, TSH, electrolytes, serum calcium, serum glucose

b. Are there any additional investigations you could order?

BUN, Cr, ESR, vitamin B_{12} and folate, drug/toxin screen, serum lipids and cortisol, heavy-metal levels, ammonia, arterial blood gases, carotid dopplers, chest x-ray, EKG, EEG, lumbar puncture, mammography, serology for syphilis and HIV

c. When would a head CT be useful?

A head CT scan should be completed if one or more of the following are present:
i.   Age <60
ii. Rapid (over 1–2 month) decline in cognition or function
iii. Recent significant head trauma
iv. Unexplained neurological symptoms (e.g., headaches, seizures, reduced level of consciousness, localizing focal deficits)
v.   History of cancer (especially those cancers that metastasize to brain)
vi. Use of anticoagulants or history of bleeding disorder
vii. History of urinary incontinence and gait disorder (suggestive of normal pressure hydrocephalus)
viii. Gait disturbance

Evaluation: History and Physical Examination for Eating Disorders

INSTRUCTIONS FOR CANDIDATE

As a pediatric resident in a teen clinic, you are about to see Brandy, a 15-year-old adolescent. Her past medical history is unremarkable, and vaccinations are current. In familiarizing yourself with her chart, you notice that the last resident to see this patient had concerns about her falling weight and amenorrhea for the last six months. Perform a directed history and physical examination.

EVALUATION CRITERIA

I. **History**

i. **Weights**
❑ Previous Highest Weight
❑ Previous Lowest Weight
❑ Present Weight
❑ Time Frame of Weight Changes

ii. **Associated Features**
❑ Body Image
❑ Self-Induced Vomiting
❑ Use of Laxatives
❑ Use of Diuretics
❑ Episodes of Binge Eating

iii. **Associated Symptoms**
❑ Dizziness
❑ Hair Loss
❑ Palpitations
❑ Oral/Genital Ulcers
❑ Constipation
❑ Cold Intolerance/Raynaud's Phenomenon

iv. **Risk Factors for Eating Disorders**
❑ Depression/Suicidal Ideation
❑ Recent Major Losses
❑ Hx of Sexual Abuse
❑ Smoking
❑ Family Hx of Eating Disorders

    v. **Medical History**
- ❏ Dietary Hx
- ❏ Exercise Hx
- ❏ Menstrual Hx
- ❏ Home/School/Employment Hx/Criminal Activity
- ❏ Previous Admissions/Surgeries/Illnesses
- ❏ Use of Alcohol, Drugs, and Tobacco

II. Physical Examination

i. General Inspection
- ❏ Height and Weight (growth plot, +/– BMI)

ii. Vital Signs
- ❏ Heart Rate
- ❏ Respiration Rate
- ❏ Postural Blood Pressure
- ❏ Temperature of Core and Extremities

iii. Appearance Changes
- ❏ Dry Skin
- ❏ Bruising
- ❏ Lanugo Hair
- ❏ Hair Loss
- ❏ Parotid Gland Enlargement
- ❏ Oral and Nasal Mucosa
- ❏ Degree of Muscle Wasting
- ❏ Sexual Maturation Stage/Genital Ulcers
- ❏ Pitting of Nail Beds
- ❏ Reflexes

III. Process Evaluation*

i. Interpersonal Skills
- ❏ Was aware of patient's nonverbal cues and emotional content
- ❏ Used reflection, checked accuracy of understanding

ii. Information Gathering
- ❏ Asked one question at a time and avoided jargon
- ❏ Used both open-ended and directed questions
- ❏ Clarified and summarized appropriately
- ❏ Ensured that patient understood questions asked
- ❏ Ensured that patient's concerns were addressed and closed interview

*See Global Process Evaluation Criteria (page 10) for a complete evaluation of the interview process.

POST-ENCOUNTER PROBES

Q1. Describe what labs you would run on a suspected eating disorder patient.

Electrolytes and venous blood gases, BUN, creatinine, liver function and enzyme tests, serum proteins

Q2. Name two common eating disorders.

Anorexia nervosa and bulimia nervosa

Q3. a. Name the psychiatric eating disorder associated with the misuse of laxatives.

Bulimia nervosa

b. If you suspected this disorder, what three clinical features could confirm your suspicions?

Any three of the following: hypothermia, bradycardia, arrhythmias, dry skin, lanugo, hair loss, scars or calluses on the dorsum of hand, loss of dental enamel, large parotid glands, pedal edema

Evaluation: History and Physical Examination of Hand Trauma

INSTRUCTIONS FOR CANDIDATE

You are the family physician in a small town, and during your busy clinic, Mr. Guirrel comes to your office with a laceration to his hand. Perform a directed history and physical examination.

EVALUATION CRITERIA

I. History
- ❏ Hand Dominance
- ❏ Occupation
- ❏ Mechanism of Injury:
- ❏   Time and Place of Injury
- ❏   Position of Hand During Injury
- ❏   Direction/Duration/Magnitude of Force
- ❏ Previous Hand Trauma/Surgeries
- ❏ Last Tetanus Immunization
- ❏ Allergies
- ❏ Complicating Conditions (e.g., arthritis/Raynaud's disease)
- ❏ Past Medical Conditions and Medications
- ❏ Last Meal (in case of immediate surgery)

II. Physical Examination

  i. Neurological

    Extrinsic Motor
- ❏ Flexion of DIP of Index Finger (median nerve)
- ❏ Flexion of DIP of 5th Digit (ulnar nerve)
- ❏ Extension of Wrist and Thumb (radial nerve)

    Intrinsic Motor
- ❏ Abduction of Thumb (median nerve)
- ❏ Abduction of Index Finger (ulnar nerve)

    Sensory
- ❏ Radial Aspect of Index Finger Pad (median nerve)
- ❏ Ulnar Aspect of 5th Digit Pad (ulnar nerve)
- ❏ Dorsum Webspace of Thumb (radial nerve)
- ❏ Individual Digital Nerves Assessment (radial and ulnar aspects by 2-pt discrimination)

  ii. Vascular
- ❏ Skin Changes (bruising/bleeding)

❏   Decreased Digital Capillary Refill
❏   Decreased Temperature
❏   Positive Allen's Test

     iii. **Tendon Palpation**
         Flexor Tendons: Passive ROM
❏   MCP — Flexion at MCP (intrinsics)
❏   PIP — Flexion at PIP (flex. dig. superficialis)
❏   DIP — Flexion at DIP (flex. dig. profundus)

         Extensor Tendons: Passive ROM
❏   MCP — Extension at MCP (communis)
❏   PIP — Extension at PIP (lat. bands of ext. dig.)
❏   DIP — Extension at DIP (lat. bands of intrinsics)

     iv. **Bones**
❏   Deformity (shortening, rotation, or scissoring of digits)

POST-ENCOUNTER PROBES

Q1. a. What are Kanavel's signs of acute suppurative tenosynovitis?
•   Tenderness of flexor tendons
•   Pain with extension
•   Edema (e.g., fusiform edema of digits)
•   Position of digits (fixed flexion)

     b. What is the management of flexor tendon sheath infections?
OR incision and drainage, irrigation, and systemic antibiotics

Q2. Human and animal bites of the hand cause infection.
     a. Name the most likely organisms involved.
Human Bites — *Eichenella*

Animal Bites — *Pasteurella multocida*

     b. Describe the first three steps in the management of bites.
Copious irrigation of open wound site(s), antibiotic therapy (clavulin), secondary closure

     c. What are the risk factors for infection?
Puncture wounds, crush injuries, wounds >12 h old, hand or foot injuries, joint injuries, patients >50 y old, immunocompromised, prosthetic joints or valves

Q3. What are the potential etiologies of Dupuytren's contracture?
Idiopathic, alcoholism, diabetes, repetitive trauma, liver disease

Q4. Describe the classic deformities of a hand affected by rheumatoid arthritis.
•   Ulnar deviation of MCPs
•   Swan-neck deformities (extension at PIP with flexion at DIP)
•   Boutonniere deformities (flexion at PIP with extension at DIP)

Evaluation: History and Physical Examination for Meningitis

INSTRUCTIONS FOR CANDIDATE

While you are working in the Emergency Room in a community hospital, Mrs. Montgomery brings in her 18-year-old daughter Stephanie because she has had a fever, new rash, and a worsening headache for the last 2 days. Perform a directed history and physical examination.

EVALUATION CRITERIA

I. **History**

    i. **Increased Intracranial Pressure**
- ❏ Headache
- ❏ Irritability
- ❏ Confusion
- ❏ Seizures
- ❏ Visual Changes
- ❏ Nausea
- ❏ Vomiting

    ii. **Meningeal**
- ❏ Photophobia
- ❏ Neck Stiffness
- ❏ Rigor
- ❏ Myalgia
- ❏ Diaphoresis

    iii. **Risk Factors**
- ❏ Low Socioeconomic Status
- ❏ Malnutrition
- ❏ Head Injury (esp. basal skull fracture <2 wks)
- ❏ Sinusitis
- ❏ Mastoiditis
- ❏ Otitis media
- ❏ Endocarditis
- ❏ Immunosuppression (carcinoma, AIDS, splenectomy, sickle-cell disease)
- ❏ Pneumonia
- ❏ CSF Shunts

II. Physical Examination
i. Increased Intracranial Pressure
❑   Bradycardia
❑   Elevated Blood Pressure
❑   Papilledema

ii. Meningeal
❑   Stiff Neck with Passive Motion
❑   Chin toward Chest
❑   Kernig's Sign*
❑   Brudzinski's Sign**

* Kernig's sign: Pain and resistance on passive knee extension when hips fully flexed.
** Brudzinski's sign: Abrupt neck flexion in the supine patient resulting in involuntary flexion of the hips and knees.

POST-ENCOUNTER PROBES

Q1. a. What is the key test to diagnose bacterial meningitis?
Lumbar puncture (LP)

    b. What are the contraindications to this test?
Signs of increased intracranial pressure

Q2. What subgroups of patients may not manifest many of the classical signs and symptoms of bacterial meningitis?
Neonates, elderly

Q3. Name three bacterial etiological agents of bacterial meningitis.
Haemophilus influenzae, Streptococcus pneumoniae, Neisseria meningitidis, Group B streptococci, *Listeria monocytogenes*

Q4. What are the most common bacterial etiological agents in children, older adults, and the elderly or immunosuppressed?
Children — *H. influenzae* if less than 4 years of age and unvaccinated; *N. meningitidis* (meningococcus)

Older adults — *Streptococcus pneumoniae* (pneumococcus)

Elderly/Immunosuppressed — *Pneumococcus, Listeria, Mycobacterium tuberculosis*, gram-negative organisms, *Cryptococcus neoformans*

Q5. Give the differential diagnosis of meningitis.
•   Acute infection of any kind
•   Acute encephalitis
•   Subarachnoid hemorrhage

Evaluation: History and Physical Examination for Obesity

INSTRUCTIONS FOR CANDIDATE

Mrs. Liza Goldsmith is a 40-year-old small-business owner who is coming to you, her family physician, with concerns over her weight. Since the start of her business two years ago, she has been keeping very long hours and not exercising. She reports a weight gain of 35 pounds over these two years. Perform a directed history and physical examination.

EVALUATION CRITERIA

I. **History**

  i. **Dietary and Body Habitus History**
- ❏ Food Preferences
- ❏ Eating Habits (no. of meals, snacks, timing of meals, etc.)
- ❏ Minimum/Maximum Weights
- ❏ Current Weight, Height, Waist Measurements
- ❏ Previous Weight Gains/Losses
- ❏ Previous Diet Attempts (types, frequency)
- ❏ Hx of Other Weight Reduction Interventions

  ii. **Exercise History**
- ❏ Current Activities (type, intensity, duration, frequency)

  iii. **Family History**
- ❏ Family Hx of Obesity
- ❏ Family Hx of Obesity-Related Co-morbidities (HTN, CAD, PVD, CVD, gallstones, diabetes, etc.)

  iv. **Medical History**
- ❏ Illnesses (e.g., Cushing's Disease, PCOD, hypothalamic injury)
- ❏ Medications (e.g., OCP, antipsychotics, antiepileptics, antidepressants)
- ❏ Alcohol Use
- ❏ Smoking

  v. **History of Obesity-Related Complications**
- ❏ Cardiovascular (e.g., HTN, CAD, CHF, PVD, CVA, arrhythmia)
- ❏ Respiratory (e.g., SOB, sleep apnea, infections, PE)
- ❏ Gastrointestinal (e.g., gallbladder disease, GERD, fatty liver)
- ❏ Musculoskeletal (e.g., osteoarthritis)
- ❏ Endocrine (e.g., Type II DM, hyperlipidemia, hyperuricemia, PCOD, hirsutism, infertility, irregular menses)

□   Neoplastic (e.g., endometrial, breast, prostate, colorectal cancers)

II. Physical Examination
i. Body Habitus Baselines
□   Weight
□   Height
□   Calculate BMI
□   Waist Circumference

ii. General
□   Vitals (PR, RR, BP)

□ ### iii. Baseline Respiratory Exam

□ ### iv. Baseline Cardiovascular Exam

POST-ENCOUNTER PROBES

Q1. Describe an effective plan to reduce weight safely for an obese patient.

A combination of the following therapies is effective in safely reducing and maintaining weight loss:

Dietary Therapy — a diet low in calories and fat content planned to achieve a deficit of 500–1000 kcal/d for a weight loss of 0.5–1 kg (1–2 lb) per week

Physical Activity — can help lose a moderate amount of weight and may help maintain that loss. Central obesity is reduced and cardiovascular fitness is improved. At the onset of weight loss, moderate-intensity physical activity for 30–45 minutes 3–5 days/week should be attempted and eventually increased to 7 days/week.

Behavioural Therapy — an adjunctive treatment for weight loss, it has its usefulness in both achieving and maintaining weight reduction.

Pharmacotherapy — useful in obese patients with BMI >30 who are otherwise healthy, or in people with BMI >27 with concomitant obesity-related risk factors or diseases. It should always be used concomitantly with other weight-loss therapies, and its continued use should be reassessed after one year. Antilipase agents such as orlistat are mildly to moderately effective.

Surgery — useful in severely obese patients (BMI >40, or >35 with co-morbid conditions) who are recalcitrant to other treatment measures. Surgical therapies, such as gastroplasty, should be used as a last resort.

Q2. Obesity can affect several organ systems, including the heart. Describe five EKG changes common to obese patients.
i.   Leftward shift of P-waves, T-waves, and QRS complexes
ii.   Low QRS voltages

iii. Left ventricular hypertrophy
iv. Left atrium hypertrophy
v. Flattening of T-waves in the inferior and lateral leads

Q3. What measurements should be used to follow the initial evaluation, management, and progress of obese patients?

- Body mass index (BMI) can be used to classify overweight and obese individuals with respect to their risk of associated diseases as compared to normal-weight individuals of the same height.
- Body weight is useful in following weight loss and efficacy of treatment regimes.
- Waist circumference is useful in the assessment of abdominal fat content. A waist circumference >88 cm (35 in) in women or >102 cm (40 in) in men is considered abnormal.

Q4. a. Identify three advantages of weight loss.

i. Lowers elevated blood pressure
ii. Improves lipid profiles (lowers total cholesterol, LDL, and triglycerides, and increases HDL)
iii. Lowers elevated blood glucose levels and reduces insulin resistance

b. Identify four disadvantages of weight loss.

i. Hypovitaminosis due to a reduction of food intake can occur.
ii. Initial weight loss may require adjustments in dosing of medications such as insulin. Improvements in blood sugar levels and insulin resistance may predispose a diabetic to hypoglycemia if insulin dosing is not adjusted.
iii. Rapid weight loss can predispose individuals to gallstones. Middle-aged females are especially at risk.
iv. Rebound weight gain can occur once dieting is stopped. This is the reason that maintenance of effective weight reduction requires changes in behaviour.

Q5. What are the medical complications of severe obesity (BMI >40)?

Sudden death, obstructive sleep apnea, CHF, nephrotic syndrome, renal vein thrombosis, immobility, Pickwickian syndrome (somnolence, polycythemia, daytime hypoventilation, cor pulmonale)

Evaluation: History and Physical Examination for Peripheral Vascular Disease

INSTRUCTIONS FOR CANDIDATE

As Mr. Morrota is leaving your office after his yearly check-up, he tells you that he forgot to mention that over the last 5 months a pain in his calves has been occurring more frequently. A year ago he could walk more than five blocks, and now he can walk only two blocks before the pain starts. Perform a directed history and physical examination.

EVALUATION CRITERIA

I. History

    i. Intermittent Claudication

❏   Location
❏   Timing (duration, onset, course)
❏   Character (quality, quantity)
❏   Severity
❏   Palliating/Provoking Factors
❏   Reproducible Pain

    Pregangrenous
❏   Night Pain
❏   Rest Pain
❏   Paresthesia (esp. in toes)

    ii. Disability Assessment/Quality of Life

❏   Impotence
❏   Impairment of ADLs and IADLs

    iii. Risk Factors for Claudication

❏   Smoking History (type, amount, duration)
❏   Diabetes
❏   Hypertension
❏   Hyperlipidemia
❏   Previous Strokes or MI

II. Physical Examination

    i. Inspection of Limbs and Skin
    Limbs
❏   Size
❏   Symmetry
❏   Edema
❏   Muscle Atrophy

Skin
- ☐ Colour/Pigmentation
- ☐ Texture
- ☐ Loss of Hair on Toes
- ☐ Ulcers/Scars
- ☐ Gangrene
- ☐ Nails (colour, texture)
- ☐ Venous Distribution (engorgement, varicosities)

ii. Palpation
- ☐ Temperature (compares both limbs)
- ☐ Capillary Refill (compares both limbs)
- ☐ Edema (compares both limbs)
- ☐ Pulses (rate, rhythm, amplitude, waveform)
- ☐ (Examined: carotid, radial, brachial, abd. aorta; renal, femoral, popliteal, dorsalis pedis, tibial)
- ☐ Pitting Edema

iii. Auscultation
- ☐ Bruits (carotid, abd. aorta, renal, iliac, femoral)

iv. Special Manoeuvres
- ☐ Leg Elevation for Pallor
- ☐ Dependency Test for Dusky Rubor

POST-ENCOUNTER PROBES

Q1. Compare and contrast arterial insufficiency verses venous insufficiency.

	Arterial Insufficiency	Venous Insufficiency
Location	• toes, points of traumas on feet and lateral malleolus	• sides of ankles esp. medial malleolus
Pain	• intermittent claudication and rest pain	• none to aching pain on dependency
Pulses	• decreased or absent	• normal
Colour	• pale (esp. on elevation) and dusky red on dependency	• normal to cyanotic (esp. on dependency) and brown pigmented with chronicity
Temperature	• cool	• normal
Edema	• absent or mild	• present and often marked
Skin changes	• thin, atrophic, shiny, hairless over toes and feet, nails thickened and ridged	• brown pigmentation, stasis dermatitis, thickening of skin, and narrowing of leg as scarring develops
Gangrene	• may develop	• does not develop

Q2. a. What is deep vein thrombosis (DVT)?

The formation of a blood clot that occludes the return of blood via a deep leg vein

b. Describe the etiologies of a DVT that may influence your approach to the directed history and physical examination.

Causes are categorized by Virchow's triad and include stasis, hypercoagulability, and endothelial damage.

Stasis — postoperative bed rest, immobilization, right-sided heart failure, obstruction, shock

Hypercoagulability — estrogen use, pregnancy, neoplasms, tissue trauma, nephrotic syndrome, deficiency of antithrombin III, protein C or S

Endothelial Damage — venulitis, trauma

c. How might a DVT present?

The affected calf or leg may be swollen, veins distended, erythematous, warm, and tender. Tachycardia, fever, and symptoms of pulmonary emboli (dyspnea, pleuritic chest pain, and hemoptysis) are also possible.

Q3. a. Describe six characteristics that one might find in a patient suffering from acute limb ischemia.

Pain, pallor, absence of pulse, paresthesia, paralysis, and polar (cold)

b. What are some causes of acute limb ischemia?

Emboli (from cardiac or arterial source), arterial thrombosis (atherosclerosis, infection, hematologic disorders), others (arterial trauma, drug-induced vasospasm, aortic dissection)

Q4. Contrast chronic vs critical ischemia.

Chronic	Critical
• Discomfort with exertion (calves)	• Night and rest pain
• Pain relieved with rest (5–10 minutes)	• Ulcerations and gangrene
• Reproducible pain (claudication distance)	• Bruits
	• Pallor on elevation and rubor on dependency

Q5. A very serious arterial disease that a clinician would not want to miss diagnosing includes an abdominal aortic aneurysm. Describe the symptoms and signs that would indicate this condition.

Hypotension, palpable pulsatile mass (felt above umbilicus), bounding femoral pulse, pain (abdominal, flank, and back), and syncope

Evaluation: History and Physical Examination for Rheumatoid Arthritis

INSTRUCTIONS FOR CANDIDATE

In an after-hours clinic, a 34-year-old woman reveals to the intake nurse that she wants to see a family doctor about stiffness in her hands. Her name is Ode May. Perform a directed history and physical examination.

EVALUATION CRITERIA

I. History

i. Pain Symptoms
- ❏ Location of Affected Joints
- ❏ Number of Affected Joints
- ❏ Timing (onset, duration, course)
- ❏ Character (quality, quantity)
- ❏ Provoking/Palliating Factors

ii. Associated Features
- ❏ Inflammation (edema, erythema, deformity)
- ❏ Weakness
- ❏ Morning Stiffness
- ❏ Limitations in Range of Motion
- ❏ Effects on ADLs

iii. Extra-Articular Features
- ❏ Eyes (red, dry, photophobia)
- ❏ Mouth (dryness, ulcers)
- ❏ Chest (dyspnea, heart murmur)
- ❏ Extremities (skin ulcers, rashes)
- ❏ Neurologic (peripheral neuropathy)

iv. Medical History
- ❏ Medications, Allergies, and Smoking
- ❏ Hx of Major Illnesses (esp. autoimmune)
- ❏ Hospitalizations/Surgeries
- ❏ Hx of Autoimmune Illnesses

II. Physical Examination

i. General Inspection (knee, shoulder, wrist)
- ❏ Edema
- ❏ Erythema

- ❏ Deformity (enlargement of MTP, MCP, or PIP; ulnar deviation, subluxation)
- ❏ Muscle Wasting

ii. Palpation (knee, shoulder, wrist)
- ❏ Warmth
- ❏ Tenderness
- ❏ Effusion
- ❏ Crepitus
- ❏ Laxity
- ❏ Instability

iii. Range of Motion (knee, shoulder, wrist)
- ❏ Active Motion
- ❏ Passive Motion
- ❏ Stress Pain

iv. Extra-Articular Screens
- ❏ Head and Neck Lesions (red eyes, oral lesions)
- ❏ Respiratory Lesions (effusions, fibrosis)
- ❏ Cardiovascular Lesions (murmurs)
- ❏ Extremities (ulcers, rashes, calf edema)
- ❏ Neurology (peripheral neuropathy)

POST-ENCOUNTER PROBES

Q1. What is Rheumatoid Factor?

It is an IgM antibody that is directed against the Fc domain of IgG. It is not specific for RA, and 5% of healthy people are positive (10%–20% over the age of 65). It is increased in hepatitis B, SLE, and many other conditions. 1:60 is suspicious and 1:160 is positive.

Q2. Compare and contrast rheumatoid arthritis and osteoarthritis with respect to process, common locations, pattern of spread, onset, and progression and duration.

	Rheumatoid	Osteoarthritis
Process	Chronic inflammation of synovial membranes with secondary erosion of adjacent cartilage and bone, and damage to ligaments and tendons	Degeneration and progressive loss of cartilage within the joints, damage to underlying bone, and the formation of new bone at the margins of the cartilage
Common locations	Hands (PIP, MCP), feet (MCP), wrists, knees, elbows, ankles	Knees, hips, hands (DIP, sometimes PIP), cervical and lumbar spine, wrists, and joints that were previously injured or diseased

continued

	Rheumatoid	Osteoarthritis
Pattern of spread	Symmetrically additive; progresses to other joints while persisting in the initial ones	Additive; however, only one joint may be involved
Onset	Usually insidious	Usually insidious
Progression and duration	Often chronic, with remissions and exacerbations	Slowly progressive, with temporary exacerbations after periods of overuse.

Q3. What is Raynaud's disease?

Episodic spasm of the small arteries and arterioles without organic occlusion. It is aggravated by cold and emotional upset. A warm environment alleviates it. There are colour changes in the distal fingers, with the progression of severe pallor (essential for the diagnosis) followed by cyanosis and then redness. Numbness and tingling are common. The episodes are brief but recurrent. It can involve one or all of the fingers.

Q4. Compare the associated symptoms of rheumatoid arthritis and osteoarthritis under the following categories: swelling, stiffness, limitation of motion, and generalized symptoms.

	Rheumatoid	Osteoarthritis
Swelling	Frequent swelling of synovial tissue in joints or tendon sheaths; also subcutaneous nodules	Small effusions in the joints may be present, especially in the knees; also bony enlargement
Stiffness	Prominent, often for an hour or more in the mornings, also after inactivity	Frequent but brief (usually 5–10 min), in the morning and after inactivity
Limitation of motion	Often develops	Often develops
Generalized symptoms	Weakness, fatigue, weight loss, and low fever are common	Usually absent

Q5. Identify six measures useful in the management of rheumatoid arthritis.

i.   Education and counselling
ii. NSAIDs and physiotherapy
iii. Corticosteroid injections
iv. Disease-modifying agents (antimalarial, gold, methotrexate, sulfasalazine, imuran)
v.   Tumour necrosis factor inhibition—inflixamab
vi. Surgery (joint replacement or fusion)

Evaluation: History and Physical Examination for Stroke

INSTRUCTIONS FOR CANDIDATE

Mrs. Wong is a 52-year-old woman with hypertension and high blood sugar. She arrives at your walk-in clinic brought by her son because she has been experiencing weakness and numbness in her left arm intermittently for two days. Perform a directed history and physical examination.

EVALUATION CRITERIA

I. **History**

   i. **Weakness**
- ☐ Location and Extent
- ☐ Time Course (onset, duration, change with time)
- ☐ Previous Episodes (TIAs)
- ☐ Quality of Deficit (sensory, movement, power)

   ii. **Associated Symptoms**
- ☐ Paresthesia
- ☐ Pain
- ☐ Dizziness
- ☐ LOC
- ☐ Amaurosis Fugax
- ☐ Slurred Speech
- ☐ Skin Changes (colour, swelling, warmth)
- ☐ Injury or Trauma
- ☐ Infection (fever, chills, sweating)

   iii. **Risk Factors**
- ☐ Family Hx of Neurological Disease
- ☐ Hx of Stroke
- ☐ Hx of MI, Murmur, Palpitations, Rheumatic Heart Disease
- ☐ Atherosclerosis RF (hypertension, DM, FHx of CAD, hypercholesterolemia, smoking)

   iv. **Impact on ADLs**
- ☐ Is the patient R or L handed?
- ☐ Gross Motor (reaching shelves, opening doors)
- ☐ Fine Motor (buttoning shirt, using keys, writing)
- ☐ Impact on Personal and Family Life

II. Physical Examination

i. Inspection

❏ Compares right arm to left arm for:
❏   Atrophy
❏   Fasciculation
❏   Abnormal Position
❏   Abnormal Movements

ii. Tone

❏ Compares right arm to left arm for:
❏   Rigidity
❏   Spasticity (velocity dependent)

iii. Power

❏ Compares and grades right-arm to left-arm power for:
❏   Shoulder Extension and Abduction
❏   Elbow Flexion, Extension, Pronation, and Supination
❏   Wrist Flexion, Extension, Ulnar and Radial Deviation
❏   Digit Abduction, Adduction, Thumb Extension, and Thumb Opposition
❏   Pronator Drift Test

iv. Reflexes

❏ Compares and grades right-arm to left-arm reflexes for:
❏   Biceps (C5–6), Brachioradialis (C5,6), and Triceps (C7,8)

v. Coordination

❏ Finger to Nose Test
❏ Rapid Alternating Movement

POST-ENCOUNTER PROBES

Q1. Explain the difference between TIA and reversible ischemic neurological deficit (RIND).

A TIA is a stroke syndrome with neurological symptoms lasting from a few minutes to as long as 24 hours, followed by complete functional recovery. A RIND is a condition in which a person has neurological abnormalities similar to acute completed stroke, but the deficit disappears after 14 to 36 hours, leaving few or no detectable neurological sequelae.

Q2. What is amaurosis fugax?

It is transient monocular blindness due to episodic retinal ischemia, usually associated with ipsilateral carotid artery stenosis or embolism of the retinal arteries resulting in a sudden, and frequently complete, loss of vision in one eye.

Q3. What are the indications for carotid endarterectomy in stroke patients?

Carotid endarterectomy is recommended for patients with surgically accessible internal carotid artery stenoses equal to or greater than 70% of the more distal, normal lumen diameter. This recommendation assumes that: the stenosis is symptomatic (causing transient ischemic attacks, nondisabling stroke, or retinal infarction); there is no worse atherosclerotic disease distally; the patient is otherwise stable; and the rates of major surgical complications of the treating surgeon are less than 6%.

Q4. What are the indications for echocardiography in stroke patients?

Echocardiography is recommended in patients with stroke and clinical evidence of cardiac disease by history, physical examination, electrocardiography, or chest radiography.

Q5. There are different treatments for ischemic strokes, which may vary according to their etiologies. Describe three sources of strokes and their corresponding treatments.

Cardiogenic — anticoagulants (warfarin)

Atherosclerotic/Lacunar/Unknown — antiplatelet therapy (acetylsalicylic acid [aspirin], clopidogrel)

Significant Vessel Stenosis — endarterectomy

Management of risk factors, such as diabetes mellitus, dyslipidemia, hypertension, and smoking, is recommended for all conditions.

Evaluation: History and Physical Examination for Thyroid

INSTRUCTIONS FOR CANDIDATE

For 6 months, Sammy Raciborski, a 73-year-old man, has been experiencing a hoarse voice and decreased energy, and complains of solid food getting stuck when he swallows. Perform a directed history and physical examination.

EVALUATION CRITERIA

I. **History**

i. Neck Mass
❑   Location
❑   Size and Number
❑   Timing (duration, onset, course)
❑   Character (quality, quantity)
❑   Severity
❑   Pain Associated with Mass
❑   Palliating/Provoking Factors

ii. Associated Symptoms
❑   General (agitation, nervousness, heat intolerance)
❑   Eyes (double vision, difficulty with eye movement)
❑   Head and Neck (hoarseness, stridor)
❑   Cardiac (palpitations)
❑   GI (dysphagia, weight loss, incr. bowel movement)
❑   GU (polyuria, decr. fertility, decr. menses)
❑   Neurology (tremulousness, weakness, fatigue)
❑   Dermatology (thinning hair, hyperpigmentation, myxedema, diaphoresis)

iii. Medical History
❑   Medications, Allergies, and Smoking
❑   Hx of major illnesses (esp. autoimmune)
❑   Hospitalizations/Surgeries
❑   Radiation Exposure
❑   Family Hx of Multiple Endocrine Neoplasia or Medullary Cancer
❑   Family Hx of Goiter or Nodules

II. Physical Examination

i. General Inspection
❏ Location and Size of Thyroid
❏ Observation of Thyroid When Patient Swallows
❏ Exophthalmos, Lid Lag, and Lid Retraction
❏ Onycholysis
❏ Texture of Skin (fine, smooth, or velvety)
❏ Pretibial Myxedema

ii. Palpation
❏ Examines Mass (tenderness, hardness, nodularity)
❏ Heart Rate
❏ BP (notes presence/absence of incr. pulse pressure)
❏ Reflexes (hyperactive with slow relaxation)

iii. Auscultation
❏ Auscultates Thyroid for Bruits

POST-ENCOUNTER PROBES

Q1. What are the signs and symptoms of hypothyroidism?
Fatigue, cold intolerance, slowing of mental and physical performance, hoarseness, enlarged tongue, slow pulse, pericardial effusion, anorexia, weight gain, constipation, paresthesia, slow speech, muscle cramps, hung-up reflexes, menorrhagia, amenorrhea, anovulatory cycles, periorbital edema, rough skin, dry coarse hair, anemia

Q2. Give a differential diagnosis of benign and malignant thyroid nodules.
Benign Nodules — Hashimoto's thyroiditis, Hürthle adenoma, follicular adenoma, multinodular goiter

Malignant Nodules — papillary, follicular, medullary, anaplastic, 1° lymphoma, metastatic tumour of breast or kidney tumours

Q3. Identify some suggestive features of malignant nodules from:
   a. history
   b. physical exam
   c. ultrasound

History — age <30 years old or >60 years old, single nodules, history of head or neck irradiation, compressive symptoms (pain, dysphagia, stridor, hoarseness)

PE — fixed and firm solitary nodule with enlarged regional lymph nodes

Ultrasound — solitary nodule, irregular halo, hypoechoic, punctate calcification, and increased blood flow

Evaluation: History and Physical Examination for Trauma (Primary Survey)

INSTRUCTIONS FOR CANDIDATE

While you are working in the Emergency Department of a peripheral hospital, the paramedics bring in Mr. Windermeir, a 35-year-old male who was hit by a car while crossing an intersection. Perform a directed history and physical examination. Please perform only a primary survey.

[Note: This scenario is somewhat different from other OSCE scenarios, since the candidate is expected to do the history and physical examination at the same time, and at times indicate the appropriate treatment/action.]

EVALUATION CRITERIA

PRIMARY SURVEY (ABCDE)

I.   Airway Assessment
❏   Assesses Ability to Speak
❏   Assesses Ability to Breathe
❏   Looks for (or Mentions) Causes of Airway Obstruction:
❏   Apnea
❏   Noisy Breathing
❏   Respiratory Distress
❏   Failure to Speak
❏   Dysphonia
❏   Extra Sounds
❏   Agitation, Confusion (e.g., level of consciousness)
❏   Cyanosis
❏   Universal Choking Sign
❏   Looks for Facial and/or Neck Trauma
❏   Looks inside Mouth
❏   Assumes C-Spine Injury (mentions would immobilize c-spine with a collar and sand bags, if not done already)
❏   If Airway Compromised, States That Would Secure Airway by Appropriate Means (e.g., nasopharyngeal airway)
❏   States That Will Continuously Reassess Airway

II. Breathing Assessment
❏   Assesses Respiratory Rate
    States That Would Obtain:
❏   O$_2$ saturation (pulse oxymetry)

- ❏ ABG
- ❏ CXR

Looks
- ❏ Mental Status (e.g., anxiety, agitation)
- ❏ Movement of Chest (e.g., flail chest, paradoxical)
- ❏ Accessory Muscle Use
- ❏ Colour (e.g., cyanosis, pale)

Listens
- ❏ Sound of Airway Obstruction (e.g., stridor)
- ❏ Breath Sounds
- ❏ Air Entry Symmetry
- ❏ Air Escaping

Feels
- ❏ Palpation of Trachea to Assess Shift
- ❏ Chest Wall for Crepitus
- ❏ Subcutaneous Emphysema
- ❏ Flail Segments
- ❏ Sucking Chest Wounds
- ❏ Percussion of Chest

- ❏ If Breathing Compromised, States That Would Treat Appropriately (e.g., nasal prongs, venturi mask, bag-valve mask)

III. Circulation Assessment
- ❏ Assesses Pulse Rate
- ❏ Assesses Pulse Quality (strength)
- ❏ Obtains BP and Pulse Pressure
- ❏ Assesses Capillary Refill
- ❏ Assesses Skin Colour
- ❏ Asks for Urinary Output Estimation (if available)
- ❏ Stops Any Major External bleeding
- ❏ Inserts Two Peripheral Large-Bore IVs

- ❏ If Peripheral Access Difficult, States That Would Obtain Central IV Access

IV. Disability Assessment
- ❏ Assesses LOC by the AVPU method:
- ❏   Is Alert
- ❏   Responds to Verbal Stimuli
- ❏   Responds to Painful Stimuli
- ❏   Is Unresponsive
- ❏ Assesses Pupils
- ❏   Size
- ❏   Reactivity
- ❏ Assesses Extremity Movement

V. Exposure
❑ States Would Expose (undress) Patient Entirely
❑ States Would Keep Patient Warm to Avoid Hypothermia

VI. General—Asks for (if not already done):
❑ Vitals q5–15 Minutes
❑ EKG
❑ Monitors (e.g., blood pressure, pulse oxymetry)
❑ Foley Catheter (if indicated)
❑ NG Tube (if indicated)
❑ CBC, Electrolytes, BUN, Cr, Glucose, Coags., Cross & Type, HCG, Toxicology Screen, LFTs, Amylase, etc.

POST-ENCOUNTER PROBES

Q1. What are the indications for intubating a patient?
- Glasgow Coma Score ≤8
- Patient is unable to protect and maintain airway
- O_2 sat. <90% with 100% oxygen
- Inadequate spontaneous ventilations
- Profound shock
- Transfer of critically ill patients to another centre

Q2. What is the estimated systolic blood pressure if a pulse is palpable at:
a. radial artery
>80 mmHg

b. femoral artery
>70 mmHg

c. carotid artery?
>60 mmHg

Q3. a. What are the signs of a tension pneumothorax?
Observation — respiratory distress, hypotension, distended neck veins, cyanosis, asymmetry of chest wall motion

Palpation — tracheal deviation away from the pneumothorax

Percussion — percussion hyperresonance on the affected side

Auscultation — unilateral absence of breath sounds

b. How is it relieved?
Insert a large-bore angiocath or IV needle in the 2nd intercostal space midclavicular line. A chest tube should then be inserted in the 5th intercostal space, anterior axillary line.

Q4. What are some potential life-threatening injuries to the chest?

CHEST

Contusion of the heart or lungs

Hernia (traumatic diaphragmatic herniation)

ESophageal perforation

Tracheobronchial disruption or traumatic injury of the aorta

Q5. What drugs can be given through an endotrachial tube?

NAVEL: Naloxone HCl, Atropine sulphate, Ventolin (salbutamol), Epinephrine, Lidocaine hydrochloride

Q6. Name the different causes of shock.

S — Spinal/Neurogenic

H — Hypovolemic (e.g., hemorrhage)

O — Obstructive (e.g., tamponade, tension pneumothorax)

C — Cardiogenic (e.g., MI)

K — AnaphylaKtic

Q7. When a patient is in need of a blood transfusion, and you are unsure of the patient's blood type, what blood type would you transfuse?

Male — O positive

Female — O negative

Evaluation: History and Physical Examination for Trauma (Secondary Survey)

INSTRUCTIONS FOR CANDIDATE

While you are working in the Emergency Department of a major teaching centre, EMS brings in a 28-year-old patient who fell from a scaffold 4 m high. Perform a directed history and physical examination. The primary survey has already been completed. Please perform a secondary survey.

[Note: This scenario is somewhat different from other OSCE scenarios, since the candidate is expected to do the history and physical examination at the same time, and at times indicate the appropriate treatment/action.]

EVALUATION CRITERIA
SECONDARY SURVEY (ABCDE)

I. **History**
    AMPLE:
❏   Allergies
❏   Medication
❏   Past Medical Hx
❏   Last Meal
❏   Events Related to Injury
❏   If patient unresponsive, or not able to provide Hx, request from EMS, family, etc.

II. **Head and Neck**
    Assesses Pupils:
❏   Size
❏   Equality
❏   Reactivity to Light
❏   Extraocular Movements
❏   Nystagmus
❏   Fundoscopy
❏   Palpates Facial Bones and Scalp
❏   Looks at Tympanic Membranes

III. **Chest**
❏   Looks for Flail Chest
❏   Looks for Subcutaneous Emphysema
❏   Reauscultates Lung Fields
❏   Orders Chest X-Ray

IV. Abdomen

i. Inspection
- ❏ Contusion
- ❏ Abrasion
- ❏ Distention

ii. Palpation
- ❏ Guarding
- ❏ Tenderness
- ❏ Rebound or Shake Tenderness
- ❏ Rigidity

iii. Percussion
- ❏ Tenderness

iv. Auscultation
- ❏ Bowel Sounds

v. Direct Rectal Examination
- ❏ Occult or Frank Blood
- ❏ Tone
- ❏ Prostate for Male
- ❏ Bimanual Pelvic Exam for Female

vi. MSK
Examines Extremities for:
- ❏ Fractures
- ❏ Swelling
- ❏ Deformities
- ❏ Contusions
- ❏ Tenderness

States Would Log-Roll Patient and:
- ❏ Palpate C-Spine if Possible
- ❏ Palpate T-Spine
- ❏ Palpate L-Spine

For Pelvis:
Assesses Pelvic Stability in 3 Planes:
- ❏ AP
- ❏ Lateral
- ❏ Vertical
- ❏ Palpates Iliac Crests
- ❏ Palpates Symphysis Pubis

vii. Neurological
- ❏ Calculates Glasgow Coma Scale
- ❏ Performs Full Cranial Nerve Exam
- ❏ Assesses Spinal Cord Integrity
- ❏ Assesses Distal Sensation and Motor Ability

- ❏   If Pt Unconscious, Determines Response to Pain or Other Stimuli
- ❏   Looks for Signs of Incr. Intracranial Pressure:
  - ❏   Deteriorating LOC
  - ❏   Deteriorating Pattern of Breathing
  - ❏   Seizures
  - ❏   Lateralizing Signs
  - ❏   Papilledema
  - ❏   Cushing's Response (High BP, decreased HR)

POST-ENCOUNTER PROBES

Q1. a. How do you assess the Glasgow Coma Scale?

The Glasgow Coma Scale (GCS) is assessed by adding up the following scores:

Eyes Open
- Spontaneously (4)
- To voice (3)
- To pain (2)
- No response (1)

Best Verbal Response
- Answers questions appropriately (5)
- Confused, disoriented (4)
- Inappropriate words (3)
- Incomprehensible sounds (2)
- No verbal response (1)

Best Motor Response
- Obeys commands (6)
- Localizes pain (5)
- Withdraws to pain (4)
- Decorticate response (abnormal flexion) (3)
- Decerebrate response (abnormal extension) (2)
- No motor response (1)

b. What are the maximum and minimum numbers for the scale?

The maximum for the GCS is 15, and the minimum is 3.

c. How does the GCS provide an indication of the severity of injury?

A GCS of 13–15 indicates a mild injury, a GCS of 9–12 indicates a moderate injury, and a GCS <8 indicates a severe injury. However, one has to keep in mind that changes in the GCS are more important than the actual numbers.

d. If the patient is intubated, how is the GCS reported?

If a patient is intubated, one cannot assess the verbal response score. Therefore, the GCS is reported out of 10, and a T is added indicating that the patient is intubated. For example, GCS 7+T.

Q2. a. What are the contraindications to inserting a Foley catheter?

Blood at the meatus, ecchymosis of the scrotum, or a high-riding prostate on digital rectal examination

b. If any of the above are seen, how would you rule out a urethral tear or ruptured bladder?

Perform a retrograde cystourethrogram.

Q3. What is the treatment for increased ICP?

- Intubation and hyperventilation
- IV 20% mannitol at 1 g/kg
- Elevation of head of bed
- Minimizing IV fluids
- Sedation of patient
- Hypothermia (last-ditch effort)

Q4. How would you clear a C-spine with X-rays?

i. Obtain three views of the C-spine: AP, lateral C1-T1, odontoid.
ii. On the lateral, look for the ABCS:
    - Look for alignment and adequacy.
    - Check anterior vertebral line, posterior vertebral line, posterior border facets, laminar fusion line, and posterior spinous line for step-offs or discontinuity.
    - Check for maintenance of cervical lordosis.
    - Must see C7–T1 junction.
    - Look for widening of the interspinous space or facet joints.
    - Check atlanto-axial articulation.
    - Check atlanto-occipital joint.
    - Look at bones.
    - Check height, shape, and width of every vertebral body.
    - Check that all laminae, facets, and pedicles are not doubled (i.e., no rotation).
    - Check that transverse process of C7 points downward, transverse process of T1 points upward.
    - Look at cartilages.
    - Look for widening of intervertebral discs suggesting vertebral compression.
    - Look at soft tissues.
    - Check that prevertebral soft tissues not wider than 5 mm at C3–C4, or wider than 20 mm at C4–C7.

Q5. a. Name four traumatic orthopedic life-threatening injuries.

Major fractures of the pelvis, massive injuries of long bones, amputations, vascular injuries that are proximal to the elbow or knee

b. Name five traumatic orthopedic limb-threatening injuries.

- Crush injuries
- Fractures above the knee or elbow
- Open fractures
- Dislocation of the knee or hip
- Compartment syndrome

Q6. What are the signs of a basal skull fracture?

- Raccoon eyes
- Battle's sign
- Hemotympanum
- CSF rhinorrhea or otorrhea

Q7. How does the reactivity of the pupils to light help in determining the cause of a patient's decrease in level of consciousness?

- If decreased LOC and reactive pupils — there is a metabolic or structural cause.
- If decreased LOC and nonreactive pupils — there is a structural cause.

Part IV

Scenarios for Physical Examinations

Evaluation: Physical Examination to Assess Coordination

INSTRUCTIONS FOR CANDIDATE

Khalid Mustafa arrives at your family medicine office. He is 48 years old and reports that he has been tripping on his treadmill for the last month. He is otherwise in good health but is concerned about problems he is having with coordination. Perform a directed physical examination.

EVALUATION CRITERIA

I. **Physical Examination**

   i. **General**
- ❏ Nystagmus
- ❏ Speech (say "British Constitution")

     Motor
- ❏ Tremor
- ❏ Muscle Tone (cogwheel, lead pipe, hypotonia)

   ii. **Gross Motor Coordination**
- ❏ Heel to Shin Test
- ❏ Finger to Nose Test

   iii. **Fine Motor Coordination**
- ❏ Rapid Alternating Movements—Lower Extremities
- ❏ Rapid Alternating Movements—Upper Extremities

   iv. **Balance**
- ❏ Rhomberg's Test
- ❏ Pull Test

   v. **Gait**
- ❏ Normal Gait
- ❏ Toe Walking
- ❏ Heel Walking
- ❏ Tandem Gait

POST-ENCOUNTER PROBES

Q1. List some causes of cerebellar lesions.

Infectious — viral infections, prion disease (Creutzfeldt–Jakob disease)

Metabolic — hepatic encephalopathy, hypothyroidism, B_{12} deficiency, thiamine deficiency, hyperthermia

Cardiovascular — anoxia, infarction, hemorrhage

Inherited — Friedreich's ataxia, ataxia telangiectasia, Ramsay–Hunt disease

Q2. Define the following terms.

Dysmetria — inability to control one's range of motion

Dysdiadochokinesia — inability to perform rapid alternating movements

Ataxia — defective voluntary muscle coordination

Dysarthria — difficult or defective speech attributed to impairments of the tongue

Nystagmus — constant involuntary cyclical movements of the eyes

Q3. An ischemic stroke to the cerebellum would leave a patient with what physical findings?

Hypotonia, ataxia, nystagmus, dysmetria, dysdiadochokinesia, normal sensory examination, normal or reduced reflexes

Q4. What are three acute and three chronic causes of ataxia?

Acute — cerebellar hemorrhage or infarction, trauma, intoxication, migraine

Chronic — alcoholic cerebellar degeneration, hypothyroidism, hydrocephalus, chronic infection (panencephalitis, rubella, prion disease), vitamin E deficiency, paraneoplastic syndrome

Q5. Describe alcoholic cerebellar degeneration.

An ataxia that affects the trunk and gait. Upper body ataxia and dysarthria are less frequent. The affected patient's gait is broad-based and is progressive but partially reversible with abstinence. It may present as a complex called Wernicke's encephalopathy (confusion, ataxia, ophthalmoplegia of CN VI).

Evaluation: Physical Examination of Cranial Nerves

INSTRUCTIONS FOR CANDIDATE

Jason Weir, a 25-year-old male whom you are seeing for the first time in your family medicine practice, comes to your office complaining that he cannot completely close his right eye and that the right side of his face droops. Perform a directed physical examination.

EVALUATION CRITERIA

I. **Physical Examination**

    i. **Cranial Nerve I (Olfactory)**
    Sensory Functions
- ❑ Nonirritant Stimuli (vanilla, coffee, mint, etc.)

    ii. **Cranial Nerve II (Optic)**
    Sensory Functions
- ❑ Visual Acuity
- ❑ Visual Fields by Confrontation

    Reflex
- ❑ Pupillary Response
- ❑ Accommodation to Light

    Fundoscopy
- ❑ Red Reflex
- ❑ Optic Disc
- ❑ Retinal Vessels
- ❑ Retinal Lesions
- ❑ Macula

    iii. **Cranial Nerve III (Oculomotor), Cranial Nerve IV (Trochlear), and Cranial Nerve VI (Abducens)**
    Inspection
- ❑ Eye Alignment

    Motor Functions
- ❑ Extraocular Movements in 9 Cardinal Positions of Gaze
- ❑ Endpoint Nystagmus
- ❑ Saccadic Eye Movements

    Sensory Functions
- ❑ Pupillary Response (light and accommodation)

iv. **Cranial Nerve V (Trigeminal)**
   Motor Functions
❑   Open Mouth
❑   Symmetry
❑   Open Mouth against Resistance
❑   Divert Jaw against Resistance
❑   Clench Teeth

   Sensory Functions—V1, V2, and V3 Regions
❑   Pain
❑   Light Touch

   Reflex
❑   Corneal Reflex
❑   Jaw Jerk Reflex

v. **Cranial Nerve VII (Facial)**
   Inspection
❑   Asymmetry in Face

   Motor Functions
❑   Raise Eyebrows
❑   Wrinkle Forehead
❑   Close Eyes Tight
❑   Show Teeth
❑   Puff Cheeks
❑   Tense Platysma Muscle
❑   Speech—Pa Test (patient says "PAH")

   Sensory Functions
❑   Anterior $\frac{2}{3}$ of Tongue for Taste

vi. **Cranial Nerve VIII (Vestibulocochlear)**
   Sensory Functions
❑   Auditory Acuity (whisper test)
❑   Rinne Test
❑   Weber Test

vii. **Cranial Nerve IX (Glossopharyngeal) and Cranial Nerve X (Vagus)**
   Inspection
❑   Voice (hoarseness, nasality)

   Motor Functions
❑   Swallow Test
❑   Speech—Ah and Ka Test (patient says "AH" and "KAH")

   Reflex
❑   Gag Reflex

viii. Cranial Nerve XI (Accessory)
Motor Functions
- ❏ Shoulder-Shrug Test
- ❏ Rotation of Head against Resistance

ix. Cranial Nerve XII (Hypoglossal)
Inspection
- ❏ Patient's Speech (notes dysarthria)
- ❏ Atrophy
- ❏ Tongue Deviation
- ❏ Fasciculation

Motor Functions
- ❏ Tongue Pushed against Cheek Test
- ❏ Speech—Ta Test (patient says "TAH")

POST-ENCOUNTER PROBE

Q1. Identify three conditions in which the physician absolutely needs to test the olfactory nerve (CN I).

Loss of taste, frontal lobe damage, and trauma to the cribriform plate

Q2. a. What is a Marcus Gunn pupil?

A pupil that paradoxically dilates with light due to a relative pupillary afferent defect

b. What is an Argyll Robertson pupil?

A pupil that has reduced constriction to light but will constrict in an accommodation reflex. This is a clinical finding associated with syphilis.

c. What does a unilateral pupillary dilation indicate?

Herniation causing ophthalmic nerve compression

Q3. When inspecting the face during a trigeminal nerve examination, what are you looking for?

Temporal muscle wasting and lateral jaw deviation to the side of the lesion

Q4. a. Which cranial nerve is affected in Bell's palsy?

Facial nerve (CN VII)

b. What is the associated clinical finding, and how can it be distinguished from a stroke in the motor complex?

Facial paralysis on the same side of the lesion. Bell's palsy is a lower motor neuron lesion, meaning the forehead is also affected. This is in contrast to a stroke, which affects upper motor neurons, thus sparing forehead involvement.

Evaluation: Physical Examination of the Hip

INSTRUCTIONS FOR CANDIDATE

Mrs. Dimayuga slipped in the shower this morning and is complaining about left hip soreness. She is a 62-year-old woman with osteoarthritis. Her past medical history is relevant for a hysterectomy and bisalpingoophorectomy completed 12 years ago. Perform a directed physical examination.

EVALUATION CRITERIA

I. Physical Examination

i. Functional Manoeuvres
- ❏ Patient's Gait (antalgic, Trendelenburg, steppage, hemiparetic, etc.)
- ❏ Trendelenburg's Sign

ii. Inspection
- ❏ Compensatory Posture (e.g., scoliotic/flexion/abduction/adduction deformity)
- ❏ Measure of True Leg Length.
- ❏ Measure of Apparent Leg Length
- ❏ Symmetry, Deformity, Signs of Inflammation/Trauma

iii. Palpation
- ❏ Palpation of Greater Trochanter and Bursa
- ❏ Leg roll

iv. Range of Motion
- ❏ Active and Passive ROM for:
- ❏   Flexion/Extension
- ❏   Abduction/Adduction
- ❏   Internal/External Rotation

v. Special Manoeuvres
- ❏ Thomas Test

POST-ENCOUNTER PROBES

Q1. Where is pain felt in the following conditions?

Osteoarthritis — radiation of pain to groin

Bursitis — pain over the superior margin of the greater trochanter

Sacroiliitis — pain localizing to sacroiliac joint

Q2. Describe true and apparent leg lengths and what the discrepancies in these lengths suggest.

True Leg Length — distance between anterior superior iliac spine to medial malleolus. Differences in length suggest hip joint pathology.

Apparent Leg Length — distance between umbilicus and medial malleolus. Differences in length suggest a pelvic tilt, possibly resulting from adduction abnormality.

Q3. Describe compensatory postures that might be seen in an examination of the hip.

- If there is a scoliotic deformity, one may see flexion of the longer leg.
- If there is an abduction deformity, one may see flexion of ipsilateral knee.
- If there is an adduction deformity, one may see flexion of contralateral knee.
- If there is a flexion deformity, one may see an exaggerated lordosis.

Evaluation: Physical Examination for Complications of Essential Hypertension

INSTRUCTIONS FOR CANDIDATE

Mr. Lim is a 58-year-old man with a longstanding history of hypertension. In checking his chart, you see that other physicians at your clinic have documented systolic blood pressures in the 170–180 mmHg range over the last year. Today, your assistant tells you that Mr. Lim's vital signs are as follows: pulse is 76 and regular, respiration is 12, and blood pressure is 166/94. Mr. Lim is in your office at the request of the last physician to see him, who has requested an assessment of potential chronic complications of essential hypertension. Perform a directed physical examination.

EVALUATION CRITERIA

I. **Physical Examination**
    i. **Retina**
    ❑   Papilledema (blurring of disc margins, no venous pulsations)
    ❑   Narrowing/Irregularity of Arterioles
    ❑   Arterial–Venous Nicking
    ❑   Flame or Dot Hemorrhages
    ❑   Cotton-Wool Spots

    ii. **Cerebral Vasculature**
    ❑   Cranial Nerve Exam
    ❑   Motor Exam
    ❑   Sensory Exam
    ❑   Cerebellar Exam

    iii. **Central Vasculature**
    ❑   Jugular Venous Pressure (waveform, height)
    ❑   Palpation for Rate/Rhythm/Contour of Carotids
    ❑   Auscultation for Bruits of Carotids

    iv. **Cardiac**
    ❑   Palpation of PMI for Location/Size/Duration
    ❑   Palpation for Heaves/Thrills
    ❑   Auscultate Apex, Tricuspid, Pulmonic, Aortic Areas
    ❑   Auscultate for S3, S4 in LLD

v. Peripheral Vasculature
❑   Palpation for Rate/Rhythm/Contour
❑   Auscultation for Bruits in:
❑   Abdominal Aorta
❑   Renal Arteries
❑   Femoral Arteries
❑   Popliteal Arteries
❑   Posterior Tibial Artery
❑   Dorsalis Pedis Artery

vi. Fluid Status and Renal
❑   JVP Examination
❑   Sacral or Pedal Edema

POST-ENCOUNTER PROBES

Q1. Describe how a person is diagnosed with essential hypertension.

1st Visit — A high blood pressure is noted and a second measure is taken. A patient who presents with a BP >200/120 is considered to have hypertensive urgency and requires immediate management. Regardless, discuss and review the medical record for clues indicating end-organ damage (coronary artery disease, cerebral vascular disease, peripheral vascular disease, retinal disease, and renal insufficiency). Arrange for four more follow-up visits over the course of 6 months.

2nd Visit — Repeat blood pressure measurements and complete baseline investigations.

3rd Visit — Repeat blood pressure measurements. If BP is still elevated and end-organ damage is present, then a diagnosis of hypertension is made and both nonpharmacologic and pharmacologic therapies are started. If no end-organ damage is present, continue to next two visits.

4th and 5th Visits — Repeat blood pressure measurements. If the BP is elevated at the fifth visit, a diagnosis of hypertension is made and treatment should begin. If at the last visit the BP is below 140/90 and no end-organ damage is present, a diagnosis of hypertension cannot be made and the patient is reassessed at 1 year.

Q2. What are the indications for pharmacologic therapy for hypertension for adults <60 y/o and >60 y/o?

Adults < 60 y/o:
*   Elevation of systolic pressures >160 mmHg and/or diastolic pressures >90 mmHg
*   Evidence of end-organ damage or diabetes mellitus
*   Presence of other cardiovascular risk factors

Adults >60 y/o:

- Elevation of systolic pressures >160 mmHg and diastolic pressures >105 mmHg

Q3. What are the indications for echocardiography in patients with hypertension?

Hypertensive patients with signs and symptoms of left ventricular dysfunction or presence of coronary artery disease

Evaluation: Physical Examination of the Knee

INSTRUCTIONS FOR CANDIDATE

Mr. DeGeorgio is a 25-year-old competitive snowboarder who, while practising on his last run, hit a patch of ice and struck his right knee after wiping out. Perform a directed physical examination.

EVALUATION CRITERIA

I   Physical Examination

i.   Inspection
- ❏   Swelling/Effusion
- ❏   Erythema
- ❏   Atrophy of Quadriceps Muscle
- ❏   Deformity (genu valgum, genu varum)
- ❏   Skin Changes (bruising, discolouration)
- ❏   Stand and Bring Feet Together (centre of hip, knee, and ankle should be in straight line)

ii.   Palpitation
- ❏   Tenderness (along joint lines, patellar tendon, and lateral collaterals at 180° and 90°)
- ❏   Warmth (compare with skin temp. above the joint)
- ❏   Baker's Cyst in Popliteal Fossa
- ❏   Thickening or Swelling (in suprapatellar pouch and sides of patella)
- ❏   Crepitation with Flexion and Extension

iii.   Effusion
- ❏   Bulge Sign/Fluid Displacement Sign
- ❏   Balloon Sign/Fluctuation Test
- ❏   Patellar Tap

iv.   Range of Motion
- ❏   Flexion
- ❏   Extension

v.   Ligaments
- ❏   Anterior Drawer Test (anterior cruciate ligament)
- ❏   Pivot Shift Test
- ❏   Posterior Drawer Test (posterior cruciate ligament)
- ❏   Stability of Lateral and Medial Collateral Ligaments

vi.   Menisci
- ❏   Crouch Compression Test

❑   Anterior and Posterior Meniscal Lesions
❑   McMurray's Manoeuvre for Lateral and Medial Meniscus

vii. Other
❑   Examination of Both Knees
❑   Examination of Hips
❑   Examination of Ankles
❑   Gait

POST-ENCOUNTER PROBES

Q1. How does one perform a pivot shift test, and what is the purpose of the test?

Start with the knee in extension, then internally rotate the foot and apply valgus force to the knee. Look and feel for anterior subluxation of the lateral tibial condyle. Slowly flex while palpating the knee and feel for pivot, which is the tibiofemoral reduction. This test is intended to locate a torn anterior cruciate ligament.

Q2. What are common knee symptoms that are important to elicit in a history?

Locking — a spontaneous block to extension found with a torn meniscus or loose meniscal body

Pseudo-locking — restricted range of motion without mechanical block. This can be caused by arthritis or muscle spasm following injury.

Instability — may be described as "giving out." Usually associated with a torn anterior cruciate ligament, patellar subluxation, torn meniscus, or loose body

Traumatic Knee Swelling — an effusion that usually represents hemarthrosis, ligamentous injury with hemarthrosis, meniscal injury, or traumatic synovitis

Nontraumatic Knee Swelling — septic or crystalline arthritis, seronegative arthritis (Reiter's, psoriatic, inflammatory bowel disease, ankylosing spondylitis)

Q3. What is the classic presentation of septic arthritis, and what is the etiology (identify five)? Describe the synovial fluid composition for joint inflammation and a septic joint.

Classic Presentation—fever, erythema, pain, swelling, limited range of motion

Etiology — *N. Gonorrhoeae, S. aureus*, streptococci, gram-negative bacilli, *H. influenzae, S. epidermidis,* Lyme disease (*Borrelia burgdorferi*), viral, and other (*M. tuberculosis*, atypical mycobacteria, fungal infections, meningococcus)

Inflammatory — elevated WBC up to $100\,000/mm^3$, 40%–90% PMN, <40 mg/dL glucose, and >2.5 g/dL protein

Septic — elevated WBC up to $5\,000\,000/mm^3$, 40%–100% PMN, 20–100 mg/dL glucose, >2.5 g/dL protein

Evaluation: Physical Examination of Lymph Nodes

INSTRUCTIONS FOR CANDIDATE

Mr. Boliva is a 47-year-old businessman who has come to your office for his annual physical. On your history taking, he tells you that he has noticed nontender lumps in his neck and complains of increased fatigue and weight loss for the last 3 months. Perform a directed physical examination.

EVALUATION CRITERIA

I. **Physical Examination**

   i. **Inspection**
- ❏ Symmetry
- ❏ Masses
- ❏ Visible Nodes

   ii. **Palpation**
- ❏ Size
- ❏ Shape
- ❏ Delimitation
- ❏ Mobility
- ❏ Consistency
- ❏ Tenderness

   iii. **Head and Neck**
- ❏ Preauricular
- ❏ Posterior Auricular
- ❏ Occipital
- ❏ Tonsillar
- ❏ Submandibular
- ❏ Submental
- ❏ Superficial Cervical Chain
- ❏ Posterior Cervical
- ❏ Deep Cervical Chain
- ❏ Supraclavicular
- ❏ Infraclavicular

   iv. **Axillary and Arms**
- ❏ Epitrochlear
- ❏ Central Nodes
- ❏ Pectoral
- ❏ Lateral
- ❏ Subscapular

    v. Legs
- ❏   Superficial Inguinal
- ❏   Vertical
- ❏   Horizontal

POST-ENCOUNTER PROBES

Q1. What types of lymph nodes are found in normal persons?

Small, mobile, discrete, nontender

Q2. What does enlargement of a supraclavicular node suggest?

Possible metastasis from a thoracic or an abdominal malignancy, especially on the left supraclavicular node

Q3. What do tender nodes and hard or fixed nodes suggest?

Tender nodes suggest inflammation; hard or fixed nodes suggest malignancy.

Q4. How does one distinguish between a lymph node and a band of muscle or an artery?

Lymph nodes should be able to be rolled in two directions: up and down, and side to side. Neither a muscle nor an artery will pass this test.

Evaluation: Physical Examination for Parkinson's Disease

INSTRUCTIONS FOR CANDIDATE

As a medical student interested in neurology, you have decided to do an elective in a neurology clinic. Awaiting you in an examination room are Mr. and Mrs. Green. Mr. Green is coming to clinic on the urging of his wife. She has told the receptionist that her husband is in clinic today for a worsening tremor in his hands and sporadic unsteadiness when he walks. Perform a directed physical examination.

EVALUATION CRITERIA

I. **Physical Examination**
    i. **General Inspection**
    ❏   Tremor (at rest, pill rolling, 4–7 Hz)
    ❏   Rigid Tone (esp. wrist for cogwheel rigidity)
    ❏   Akinesia/Dyskinesia
    ❏   Postural Instability (stooped)
    ❏   Mask-like Face (lack of blinking, dysarthria)

    ii. **Coordination Test**
        Coarse Motor Control
    ❏   Heel from Knee to Ankle Test
    ❏   Finger to Nose Test

        Fine Motor Control
    ❏   Rapid Alternating Movements — Tapping Feet
    ❏   Rapid Alternating Movements — Thumb–Finger Opposition
    ❏   Rapid Alternating Movements — Pronate–Supinate Hands

        Posture and Gait
    ❏   Regular, Toe, Heel, and Tandem Gait Assessments
    ❏   (start hesitation, shuffling steps, loss of arm swing)

    iii. **Motor Examination**
        Inspection
    ❏   Muscle Bulk
    ❏   Fasciculation
    ❏   Muscle Tone

        Tone
    ❏   Upper Extremities
    ❏   Lower Extremities

- [ ] Asymmetry
- [ ] Graded

Power
- [ ] Upper Extremities
- [ ] Lower Extremities

Reflexes
- [ ] Upper Extremities
- [ ] Lower Extremities
- [ ] Clonus (both extremities)

iv. Sensory Examination
- [ ] Position or Vibration
- [ ] Pain or Temperature

v. Posture and Balance
- [ ] Rhomberg's Test
- [ ] Postural Instability (pull-back test)

POST-ENCOUNTER PROBES

Q1. What is the differential diagnosis for symptoms like those seen in Parkinson's disease?

Therapeutic Drugs — neuroleptics, metoclopramide

Toxins — MPTP (drug abusers), manganese, carbon disulfide, CO

Parkinsonism — progressive supranuclear palsy, Shy–Drager syndrome

Q2. Identify the different types of tremor and describe each type.

Rest Tremor — the slow, characteristic tremor of Parkinsonism. The hands have characteristic motion of pill rolling, alternating flexion/extension of fingers or hands, alternating pronation/supination of forearms.

Postural and Action (Kinetic) Tremor — a fast tremor that is seen best with arms and hands outstretched. It can be physiological, in which case it is always present and imperceptible to the eye. It can be an exaggerated physiological tremor, in which case it comes on with anxiety and sleep deprivation. It can come from withdrawal of alcohol, caffeine, or lithium. Hyperthyroidism or hypoglycemia can augment this tremor.

Essential Tremor — autosomal dominant inheritance. The patient usually complains of shaking when carrying a teacup, putting a glass to the mouth, or trying to eat soup. It can affect handwriting and voice.

Intention Tremor — seen in diseases of cerebellar outflow; worsens with alcohol. It is a tremor of limbs or head. It is worse at the endpoint of movement and is a contra-axial tremor.

Q3. Describe the pathology of Parkinson's Disease.

There is loss of dopaminergic nigrostriatal neurons in substantia nigra's zona compacta. Dopamine neurons degenerate, upsetting normal balance between dopaminergic inhibition and cholinergic excitation of striatal output (GABA) neurons. This results in relative increase in GABAergic output from striatum.

Q4. Describe the effects of pharmacologic treatments used for Parkinson's disease and give examples of each type.

All treatments are for symptomatic relief and do not address the underlying pathology. Each restores the ratio of dopamine to acetylcholine.

Anticholinergics — can control tremor symptoms but not the rigidity or bradykinesia. An example is benzhexol.

Exogenous Dopamine — improves the rigidity and bradykinesia but not the tremor. Examples include levodopa or levodopa with decarboxylase.

Dopamine Agonists — work on the D1, D2 dopamine receptors or some combination of them and are used to treat bradykinesia and rigidity when exogenous dopamine fails. Some examples are apomorphine, lisuride, pergolide, bromocriptine.

Monoamine Oxidase Inhibitors — inhibit the enzymes that break down dopamine, enhancing dopamine's effects. Selegiline is an example.

Amantadine — has an unknown mechanism of action in the treatment of Parkinson's disease.

Evaluation: Physical Examination for Pulsus Paradoxus

INSTRUCTIONS FOR CANDIDATE

Demonstrate how to test for pulsus paradoxus.

EVALUATION CRITERIA

I. Procedure

❑ Properly Positions Patient and BP Cuff
❑ Inflates Cuff beyond Systemic Pressure
❑ Slowly Reduces Pressure until Korotkoff Sounds Are Heard on Expiration Only and Then Notes Pressure
❑ Further Deflates Cuff until Sounds Are Heard on Both Inspiration and Expiration and Notes Pressure
❑ Ascertains Difference between Pressures
❑ Makes Determination of Pulsus Paradoxus Based on Measurements Taken
❑ Describes What Pulsus Paradoxus Is
❑ Describes Circumstances under Which Pulsus Paradoxus Occurs

POST-ENCOUNTER PROBES

Q1. a. Define pulsus paradoxus.

Pulsus paradoxus is defined as an inspiratory fall in systemic blood pressure >10 mmHg.

b. Explain its pathogenesis.

A high negative intrapleural pressure draws blood back into the vena cavae. Therefore, venous return to the right atrium and right ventricle is increased, causing increased filling of the right side of the heart. With the increased volume, the interventricular septum bulges into the left ventricular outflow tract, which in turn decreases the stroke volume and ultimately reduces systemic blood pressure. The higher-than-normal intrapleural pressure may also cause blood to be drawn into the pulmonary circulation from the left side of the heart, which would also decrease the stroke volume and ultimately reduce systemic blood pressure.

c. Describe the conditions under which one might expect to find pulsus paradoxus.

An exaggerated pulsus paradoxus can be found in:

Cardiac Conditions — cardiac tamponade, pericardial effusions, constrictive pericarditis

Respiratory Conditions — asthma, emphysema, and increased effort in ventilation

Evaluation: Physical Examination of the Shoulder

INSTRUCTIONS FOR CANDIDATE

Ms. Chawla is a medical student and a competitive rower. Just before winning a gold medal, she felt a sharp pain in her right shoulder followed by some mild swelling. Perform a directed physical examination.

EVALUATION CRITERIA

(For each of the sternoclavicular, acromioclavicular, glenohumeral, and scapulothoracic joints)

I. **Physical Examination**

   i. **Inspection**
- ❑ Swelling
- ❑ Erythema
- ❑ Asymmetry/Atrophy
- ❑ Deformity
- ❑ Skin Changes

   ii. **Palpation**
- ❑ Tenderness
- ❑ Temperature
- ❑ Edema
- ❑ Crepitus
- ❑ Biceps Groove
- ❑ Subdeltoid Bursa

   iii. **Range of Motion**
- ❑ Active and Passive ROM for:
- ❑   Flexion/Extension
- ❑   Abduction/Adduction
- ❑   Internal/External Rotation

   iv. **Special Manoeuvres**
- ❑ Apprehension Test

POST-ENCOUNTER PROBES

Q1. a. What is impingement syndrome?

Impingement of the supraspinatus tendon between the greater tuberosity of the head of the humerus and the undersurface of the acromion and acromioclavicular joint, often due to osteophytes under the acromion

b. What would you find on physical examination of this condition?

There is a painful arc felt between 90° and 130° of abduction, and tenderness with palpation of the rotator cuff.

Q2. a. Describe the apprehension test used to identify anterior shoulder dislocations.

A patient's affected arm is abducted and externally rotated until a look of apprehension is noted if the shoulder is dislocatable.

b. What are other useful physical signs?

Shoulder has "squared off" appearance, with reduction of internal rotation and possible loss of sensation and contraction over the lateral deltoid muscle.

Q3. a. Name four causes of posterior shoulder dislocation.

Epileptic seizures, ethanol intoxication, electrocution/electroshock therapy, encephalitis

b. Describe the mechanism causing the dislocation.

Posterior dislocation results from a force applied through the long axis of the arm when it is adducted, flexed, and internally rotated.

Q4. Name seven common conditions that affect the shoulder.

i.   Rotator cuff tendon tear
ii.   Rotator cuff tendinitis
iii. Frozen shoulder
iv.   Biceps tendinitis
v.   Impingement syndrome
vi.   Subscapular bursitis
vii. Glenohumeral osteoarthritis
viii. Acromioclavicular strain

Evaluation: Physical Examination of Volume Status

INSTRUCTIONS FOR CANDIDATE

You are an internal medicine resident who has been asked to see Mrs. Montgomery, a 95-year-old woman with congestive heart failure. The nursing staff were concerned with a dramatic swelling in both legs after it was noticed that she did not receive her diuretics yesterday. Perform a directed physical examination.

EVALUATION CRITERIA

I. **Physical Examination**

   i. **Blood Pressure Examination**
   - ❑ Checks BP While Pt Is Supine
   - ❑ Waits 2 Minutes before Next Reading
   - ❑ Checks BP of Pt Sitting and Legs Dependent/Standing
   - ❑ Identifies Orthostatic Hypotension
   - ❑ Checks HR While Pt Is Supine
   - ❑ Checks HR While Pt Is Sitting/Standing

   ii. **Jugular Venous Pressure Examination**
   - ❑ Properly Positions Patient (30° angle, head turned left)
   - ❑ Uses Tangential Lighting
   - ❑ Reads JVP on Right Side of Patient
   - ❑ Distinguishes JVP from Carotid (5 ways)
   - ❑ Makes Determination of JVP Height above Sternal Angle
   - ❑ Comments on Waveform (a wave, x descent, v wave, y descent)
   - ❑ Explains that Normal JVP Is 3–4 cm above Sternal Angle
   - ❑ Performs the Abdominojugular Reflux

   iii. **Edema Examination**
   - ❑ Checks for Dependent Pitting Edema (ankles, sacrum)
   - ❑ Checks for Ascites (fluid wave, dull shift.)

   iv. **Respiratory Examination**
   - ❑ Auscultates All Lung Lobes for Crackles

   v. **Cardiac Examination**
   - ❑ Auscultates the Heart for S3

POST-ENCOUNTER PROBES

Q1. a. Define jugular venous pressure.

JVP is defined as the pressure of the internal jugular system and is a direct assessment of the pressure in the right atrium of the heart.

b. Distinguish between the JVP and carotid waveforms.

JVP Waveform	Carotid Waveform
• Not palpable	• Palpable
• Multiple waveforms	• Single waveforms
• Soft, undulating quality	• Vigorous quality
• Obliterated by applied pressure	• Not affected by applied pressure
• Height changes on inspiration, sitting up or with Valsalva manoeuvre.	• Height not affected by inspiration, sitting up or with Valsalva manoeuvre.

Q2. a. Why are right-sided pulsations preferred over left-sided ones when reading the JVP?

Right-sided pulsations are preferred as left-sided measurements may be falsely elevated because of kinking of the innominate vein.

b. What features of the JVP does one describe in its assessment?

Height, character of waveform, and results of abdominojugular reflux

c. What is a normal range for JVP?

Normal range is 4–5 cm above the sternal angle.

Q3. a. When is the abdominojugular reflux considered abnormal?

Abnormality is indicated when there is a sustained rise in JVP >4 cm after applying abdominal pressure for a minimum of 15–30 seconds.

b. What is Kussmaul's sign, and why does it occur?

Kussmaul's sign is a paradoxical increase in the JVP on inspiration. It occurs because the heart is unable to accommodate the increase in the venous return that accompanies the inspiratory fall in intrathoracic pressure.

c. Identify a condition in which you would expect to find Kussmaul's sign.

Severe right-sided heart failure, constrictive pericarditis, restrictive cardiomyopathy

d. If you knew a person had a very elevated JVP but still wanted to evaluate the JVP pulsations, what could you do?

Use a higher elevation of the bed (>30°) until pulsations are seen.

Q4. a. Explain or demonstrate how you would examine a patient for orthostatic hypotension.

Measure BP in supine patient, then have the patient sit up with the legs down or have patient stand for 2 minutes before reassessing BP.

b. Define what is meant by orthostatic hypotension and the conditions in which you might see it.

With a change in body position, the systolic BP decreases (>15 mmHg), diastolic BP decreases (>0–10 mmHg), and/or heart rate increases (>20 bpm). Orthostatic hypotension is seen in conditions of autonomic dysfunction and volume depletion.

Part V

Special Scenarios

Evaluation: Interpretation of Abdominal X-Ray

INSTRUCTIONS FOR CANDIDATE

You are an intern doing an emergency rotation. Your staff has examined a patient who reported a 2-day history of constipation, nausea, and vomiting. For the last 24 hours, the patient, Mr. Somani, has not passed a bowel movement or flatus per rectum. You are asked to obtain abdominal films on this patient and interpret them.

EVALUATION CRITERIA

ROENTGENOGRAPH EXAMINATION

I.   General
- ❏   Obtains Patient Demographics (age, sex)
- ❏   States Types of Studies (e.g., flat plate, upright, etc.)
- ❏   States Study Date and Time
- ❏   Obtains Patient's Clinical History
- ❏   States That Would Obtain Previous Films for Comparison
- ❏   Critiques Quality of Film
- ❏   States Overall Initial Impression (e.g., any obvious abnormalities)

II.   Comments on (can be done in any order):

i.   Supraphrenic structures
- ❏   Lung Bases
- ❏   Pleural Effusions
- ❏   Consolidation
- ❏   Rib Fractures

ii.   Bones
- ❏   Inspects Lower Thoracic Spine
- ❏   Inspects Lumbosacral Vertebrae:
- ❏   Lytic or Sclerotic Lesions
- ❏   Degenerative Changes
- ❏   Inspects Pelvis
- ❏   Inspects Hips

iii. Soft tissues
- ❏   Fat Stripe
- ❏   Flank Stripe
- ❏   Psoas Muscles

iv. Solid viscera
- ❏ Liver (e.g., hepatomegaly)
- ❏ Spleen (e.g., splenomegaly)
- ❏ Kidneys (e.g., renal enlargement, stones)
- ❏ Gallbladder (e.g., calcifications)
- ❏ Pancreas (e.g., calcifications)
- ❏ Uterine Contour
- ❏ Bladder (e.g., contour, calcifications)
- ❏ For All Solid Viscera, Inspects for:
- ❏   Calcifications
- ❏   Masses
- ❏   Changes in Shape
- ❏   Changes in Size

v. Gas patterns
Intestinal Gas Patterns
- ❏ Dilatation
- ❏ Air–Fluid Levels
- ❏ Mucosal Thickening

Extraintestinal Gas Patterns
- ❏ Pneumoperitoneum
- ❏ Pneumobilia
- ❏ Portovenous Gas
- ❏ Abscess
- ❏ Intramural Gas

vi. Calcifications (if not already mentioned)
- ❏ Gallstones
- ❏ Appendicoliths
- ❏ Phleboliths
- ❏ Fecaliths
- ❏ Renal/Ureteral/Vesical Stones
- ❏ Pancreatic Calcifications

Candidate should give diagnosis (small bowel obstruction).

POST-ENCOUNTER PROBES

Q1. What size of bowel represents abnormal dilatations?
> 3 cm for small bowel; > 5 cm for large bowel

Q2. Where are gas–fluid levels normally seen?
In the gastric fundus on upright films, and sometimes in the first part of the duodenum or in the right colon.

Q3. a. Identify the three most common causes of small-bowel obstruction.

i. Adhesions and fibrous bands postsurgery
ii. Hernias
iii. Neoplasms

b. Identify some other causes.

- Gallstone ileus
- Small-bowel volvulus
- Intussusception

Q4. Identify the typical radiological findings of a small-bowel obstruction.

- Gaseous distention of multiple, centrally located loops of bowel
- Diameter of small-bowel loops >3 cm
- Short gas–fluid levels of various heights on uprights or left lateral decubitus films
- A "step-ladder" appearance of bowel

Q5. Identify the typical radiological findings of a large-bowel obstruction.

- Proximal large-bowel dilatation with little or no gas in the distal colon
- Short gas–fluid levels of various heights
- Diameter of large-bowel loops > 5 cm

Q6. What is the critical diameter of a dilated cecum at the point at which acute decompression is recommended?

9 cm

*See Appendix C: X-Rays (page 233) for examples of abdominal x-rays.

Evaluation: History from an Angry Patient

INSTRUCTIONS FOR CANDIDATE

It is an extremely busy night in the Emergency Room where you are working as a medical clerk. On this holiday weekend, the ER is jammed with more than 40 people waiting to be seen. You pull the next patient chart and proceed to the examination room, where Mr. I.M. Livid awaits you. You are greeted by an angry, explosive patient who is dissatisfied with having waited four and half hours to be seen by a doctor for a pulled muscle. Perform a directed history.

EVALUATION CRITERIA

I. Listening Strategies
❑ Behaves Calmly and Avoids Overreacting
❑ Copes with Interruptions and Time Constraints
❑ Demonstrates Empathy
❑ Allows Patient to Vent Verbally When Possible
❑ Considers Language and Cultural Barriers
❑ Ensures Patient's Understanding

II. Verbal Strategies
❑ Investigates Circumstances of Patient's Concerns
❑ Clarifies Information When Needed
❑ Redirects Patient's Challenge Questions
❑ Sets and Enforces Reasonable Limits with Patient
❑ Conveys Information with Brevity and Simplicity
❑ Develops Strategy to Address Patient's Concerns
❑ Summarizes Interview

III. Physical Strategies
❑ Respects Patient's Personal Space
❑ Ensures Patient's Privacy
❑ Uses Appropriate Body Language
❑ Keeps Nonverbal Cues Nonthreatening

IV. Control of Environment
❑ Interviews in a Safe and Controlled Environment
❑ Positions Self for Easy Egress
❑ Positions Patient for Easy Egress

POST-ENCOUNTER PROBES

Q1. Describe the techniques that may help prevent anger and frustration in a patient.

- Be consistent and provide easily understood information.
- Use empathy to help patient come to decisions about care.
- Discuss probable outcomes.
- Provide time to ask questions as well as periodic updates, if needed.
- Respect treatment plans and do not make changes without patient's consent.

Q2. What nonverbal and verbal techniques can be used in dealing with patient conflict?

- Reflect active listening and attentiveness through body language.
- Avoid invading personal space by standing off to the side of the patient at least a metre away.
- Make sure both parties have easy access to an exit. If personal safety is ever in question, a room that is monitored by security should be used, or a third party should attend.
- Control the urge to overreact and verbally respond to an eruption of negative emotions.
- Remain calm and professional.
- Redirect questions that challenge hospital policy or staff qualifications to the issues at hand.
- Keep information simple and concise.
- Consider language barriers; use other hospital staff to translate and clarify misunderstandings, if possible.

Evaluation: Breaking of Bad News

INSTRUCTIONS FOR CANDIDATE

Mr. Ravenfeather is a 65-year-old man with a 2-year history of decreased urinary flow and postvoid retention. Five weeks ago, he came to the clinic on the nearby reserve that you help serve with complaints of increasing lower back pain. You suspected prostate cancer and referred him to a local urologist for a biopsy and to arrange a bone scan for metastasis. In reading his chart, you become aware that the results show metastatic prostate cancer. Inform the patient of the results of the biopsy.

EVALUATION CRITERIA

I. Patient's Understanding/Ideas/Feelings
❏ Determines Impact of Illness on Patient (PERCEPTION)

II. Telling the News
❏ Determines Whether Patient Wants to Hear News (INVITATION)
❏ Prepares Patient Before Breaking Bad News
❏ Provides Dx in a Straightforward Manner
❏ Keeps Information Simple and Avoids Medical Jargon
❏ Assesses Patient's Understanding (KNOWLEDGE)
❏ Assesses Patient's Emotional State (EXPLORATION)
❏ Reiterates the Main Points
❏ Does Not Minimize or Trivialize Condition

III. Chronic Effects on Patient
❏ Changes in IADLs and ADLs.
❏ Coping Strategies
❏ Social Supports (family, friends, support groups)
❏ Concerns (loss of control, alienation, pain, mortality, sense of mutilation)
❏ Effects of Illness on Family, Social Situation, and Work
❏ Feelings of Inadequacy
❏ Risk of Substance Abuse
❏ Risk of Suicide

IV. Management and Control
❏ Assesses Current Medications and Treatments
❏ Assesses Current Rehabilitation Strategies
❏ Assesses Current Homecare Assistance

- ❏ Considers Past Hospitalizations, Treatments, and Surgeries
- ❏ Assesses Compliance with Treatments and Complications

POST-ENCOUNTER PROBES

Q1. What is the acronym used by many clinicians to describe the important features of how to break bad news?

SPIKES

Setting — use appropriate physical space and positioning, appropriate body language and eye contact, and active listening skills such as pausing, silence, nodding, smiling, repetition, clarifying, etc.

Perception — ask the patient what she or he understands, suspects, or knows about the current medical condition.

Invitation — ask whether the patient wants to know the details of the condition (not everyone will).

Knowledge — align yourself with the patient by using language he or she will understand; provide the information in small amounts, and check patient's understanding regularly.

Exploration and Empathy — identify the emotions expressed and their sources.

Strategy and Summary — think what is best medically, assess the patient's expectations of treatment, etc., propose a strategy, and agree on plan. Summarize the important issues.

Q2. (Choose the best answer.) If asked questions for which you do not have an answer, what should you do?

   a. Change the subject and ignore the initial question.

   b. Make something up, as the patient is likely to forget the information anyway, given present emotional state.

   c. Tell the patient that you do not know the answers; acknowledge patient's concerns, and explain how you will obtain answers in the near future.

   d. Make light of the patient's concerns.

(Correct answer is c.)

Q3. Patients with life-threatening illnesses and their families often suffer from grief. Describe the classic stages of grief, which might help you treat these patients and their families.

i.   Patient attempts to limit awareness of condition (shock, denial, and isolation).
ii. Patient has awareness and emotional release.
iii. Patient experiences depression.
iv. Patient has acceptance and resolution.

Q4. Identify three feelings that many grieving people experience.

- Anger
- Hopelessness
- Guilt
- Worthlessness

Q5. Identify three tasks of bereavement.

i. Accepting the reality of loss
ii. Working through the pain of grief
iii. Adjusting to life without the deceased

Evaluation: Interpretation of Chest X-Ray

INSTRUCTIONS FOR CANDIDATE

You are an intern doing an emergency rotation. Your staff has examined an elderly patient, Mr. Ryan, who reports a 3-day history of productive cough and fever. You are asked to obtain a PA and lateral chest x-ray on this patient and to interpret them.

EVALUATION CRITERIA

ROENTGENOGRAPH EXAMINATION

I. General
- ❏ Patient Demographics (age, sex)
- ❏ States Types of Studies (PA and lateral)
- ❏ States Study Date
- ❏ Obtains Patient's Clinical History
- ❏ States That Would Obtain Previous Films for Comparison
- ❏ Critiques Quality of Film:
- ❏   Patient Rotation
- ❏   Film Exposure
- ❏   Patient's Inspiration
- ❏ States Overall Initial Impression (i.e., any obvious abnormalities)

II. PA Film
Comments on (can be done in any order):

i. Bones and Joints (looking for fractures, arthritis, etc.)
- ❏ Anterior and Posterior Ribs
- ❏ Spine (vertebral columns)
- ❏ Clavicles
- ❏ Scapulae

ii. Soft Tissues (calcifications, subcutaneous emphysema, etc.)
- ❏ Axillae
- ❏ Breast Shadows (e.g., mastectomy)

iii. Pleura
- ❏ Fissures (major and minor)
- ❏ Costovertebral Angles

iv. Diaphragm
- ❏ Level
- ❏ Identifies Right and Left

- ❏ Looks for Abdominal Free Air
- ❏ Points Gastric Air Bubble

v. Heart
- ❏ Size (states that shouldn't be >50% the size of the cardiothoracic ratio)
- ❏ Looks for Calcifications
- ❏ Looks for Atrial/Ventricular Enlargement

vi. Mediastinum
- ❏ Size (in relation to cardiothoracic ratio)
- ❏ Shape
- ❏ Position of:
- ❏   Trachea
- ❏   Aortic Arch
- ❏   Right Heart Border

vii. Hila
- ❏ Size
- ❏ Compares Right and Left
- ❏ Displacement (upward/downward)

viii. Lung Parenchyma
- ❏ Looks for:
- ❏ Nodules
- ❏ Changes in Parenchymal Density
- ❏ Vascular Abnormalities (e.g., redistribution)

III. Lateral Film
Comments on (can be done in any order):

i. Bones and Joints (looking for fractures, arthritis, etc.)
- ❏ Spine (vertebral columns)
- ❏ Sternum

ii. Pleura
- ❏ Fissures (major and minor)
- ❏ Costovertebral Angles

iii. Diaphragm
- ❏ Level
- ❏ Identifies Right and Left
- ❏ Looks for Abdominal Free Air
- ❏ Points out Gastric Air Bubble
- ❏ Looks for Depression/Elevation

iv. Mediastinum
- ❏ Size (in relation to cardiothoracic ratio)
- ❏ Shape

- ❏ Position of:
- ❏   Trachea
- ❏   Aortic Arch
- ❏ Looks for Masses

v. Hila
- ❏ Size
- ❏ Compares Right and Left
- ❏ Displacement (upward/downward)

vi. Lung Parenchyma
- ❏ Looks for:
- ❏   Nodules
- ❏   Changes in Parenchymal Density
- ❏ Looks at:
- ❏   Retrosternal Clear Space
- ❏   Retrocardiac Clear Space

The candidate should give a diagnosis (left lower-lobe pneumonia).

POST-ENCOUNTER PROBES

Q1. Name the bronchopulmonary segments of the right lung.
- Right upper lobe (apical, anterior, posterior)
- Right middle lobe (medial, lateral)
- Right lower lobe (superior, lateral basal, anterior basal, posterior basal)

Q2. a. What is the silhouette sign?

The silhouette (or better, the "loss of silhouette") sign refers to the loss of the normally appearing interfaces or profiles that imply solid changes (e.g., consolidation, atelectasis) in the adjacent lung.

b. Give examples of some silhouette signs.

RML consolidation — loss of right heart border

Lingula consolidation — loss of left heart border

Anterior segment of left upper lobe — loss of aortic arch

Q3. Name four features that allow you to differentiate between the left and right hemidiaphragms in a lateral film.
- i. The right hemidiaphragm is usually higher than the left.
- ii. The left hemidiaphragm is silhouetted out by the heart.
- iii. The gastric air bubble is below the left hemidiaphragm.
- iv. The right ribs are usually magnified since they are farther away from the film than the left ribs, so the right hemidiaphragm is the hemidiaphragm that meets the right ribs.

Q4. a. What is air-space disease?

Air-space disease refers to a pathological process affecting primarily the alveoli.

b. What are the radiological findings of air-space disease?

Acinar shadows, air bronchograms, silhouette sign

c. Give a differential diagnosis for this condition.

Fluid (e.g., pulmonary edema), pus (e.g., pneumonia), cells (e.g., lung cancer), blood (e.g., hemorrhage), proteins (e.g., alveolar proteinosis)

Q5. a. What is insterstitial disease?

Interstitial disease refers to a pathological process affecting primarily the interstitium of the lung.

b. What are the radiological findings for interstitial disease?

Can have a reticular pattern (net-like), a nodular pattern (nodules), or both.

c. Give a differential diagnosis for this condition.

Pulmonary edema, miliary tuberculosis, pneumoconiosis, sarcoid

Q6. When you are interpreting a PA chest x-ray, you think you see a nodule in the apex, but the right clavicle and first rib hinder visualization. What type of chest x-ray should you get?

An apical lordotic view, which projects the first ribs and the clavicles above the lung apices

*See Appendix C: X-Rays (page 233) for examples of chest x-rays.

Evaluation: History of Chronic Disease

INSTRUCTIONS FOR CANDIDATE

Mrs. Thorossoulis is a 45-year-old woman. She has a problem with obesity and osteoarthritis in her knees and hips. Today, she comes to your clinic wanting to discuss the effects of her ailments on her quality of life. Perform a directed history.

EVALUATION CRITERIA

I. Description of Illness
- [ ] Age of Onset of Illness
- [ ] Description of Onset of Illness
- [ ] When the Disease Had the Greatest Impact
- [ ] Current Stage of Illness
- [ ] Recent Changes in Illness
- [ ] Assessment of Patient's Understanding of Illness Including Stages, Time Course, and Prognosis

II. Chronic Effects on Patient
- [ ] Changes in IADLs and ADLs
- [ ] Coping Strategies
- [ ] Social Supports (family, friends, support groups)
- [ ] Concerns (loss of control, alienation, pain, mortality, sense of mutilation)
- [ ] Effects of Illness on Family, Social Situation, and Work
- [ ] Feelings of Inadequacy
- [ ] Risk of Substance Abuse
- [ ] Risk of Suicide

III. Management and Control
- [ ] Assesses Current Medications and Treatments
- [ ] Assesses Current Rehabilitation Strategies
- [ ] Assesses Current Homecare Assistance
- [ ] Assesses Past Hospitalizations, Treatments, and Surgeries
- [ ] Assesses Compliance with Treatments and Complications

POST-ENCOUNTER PROBES

Q1. Name five common chronic conditions for which the physician might consider asking the above questions.

Diabetes, CHD, COPD, cystic fibrosis, cancer, rheumatoid arthritis, alcoholism, depression, schizophrenia, HIV/AIDS, renal failure, inflammatory bowel disease, Parkinson's disease, Alzheimer's disease, epilepsy

Q2. Name four areas in which a chronic illness may most affect the life of a teenager or young adult.

Self-confidence, peer relationships, involvement in extracurricular activities, school performance

Q3. Describe five fears often mentioned by patients with chronic illnesses such as cancer.

i.   Distance — fears associated with interpersonal changes
ii. Dependency — fears that the illness will lead to a state of helplessness
iii. Disability — fears that goals are no longer achievable
iv. Disfigurement — fears that the illness will scar or disfigure
v.   Death — fears of death and thus the illness as a source of loss

Q4. Describe what is meant by ADLs and IADLs.

ADL
- Transfers out of bed
- Going to the toilet
- Eating
- Dressing
- Getting around the home

IADL
- Banking
- Shopping
- Keeping appointments
- Travelling
- Cleaning

Evaluation: History to Evaluate Competency in Medical Decision Making

INSTRUCTIONS FOR CANDIDATE

Mrs. Geschick is a 69-year-old woman who has survived her husband for more than 10 years. She has no other family or close personal friends. Recently, she presented to the Emergency Room with chest pain. The investigations in the ER revealed a small septal myocardial infarction. During her admission, a stress test was done and was positive. Her attending cardiologist wants to complete coronary angiography with possible stenting, but Mrs. Geschick refuses and states that she is "alone in this world" and wants "to rejoin her husband." The cardiologist has asked your service, psychiatry, to assess her competency, as there have been times in the admission when she seemed confused and withdrawn. Perform a directed history to assess this patient's competency in making her own medical decisions.

EVALUATION CRITERIA

I. **History**

i. **Assessment of the Understanding of Illness**

❏ Describes the Patient's Disease Process and Assesses Patient's Understanding of the Following:

❏ Nature and Probable Outcome of the Disease

❏ Current Stage and Time Course of the Disease

❏ Course of the Disease

ii. **Assessment of the Understanding of the Proposed Management of the Disease**

❏ Describes the Proposed Management of the Disease Process and Assesses Patient's Understanding of the Following:

❏ Nature of the Proposed Treatment

❏ Alternatives to the Proposed Treatment

❏ Consequences of Accepting/Rejecting the Proposed Treatment

❏ Risks and Benefits of Each Option (including no treatment)

iii. **Assessment of the Appreciation of the Disease and Its Management**

❏ Assesses Patient's Acknowledgment of the Disease

❏ Demonstrates Patient's Understanding of Consequence of Treatment Options

❏ Determines Patient's Decision for Treatment

❏ Comments on Patient's Adherence to Decision

    i. Interpersonal Skills

❏   Was aware of patient's nonverbal cues and emotional content
❏   Used reflection, checked accuracy of understanding

    ii. Information Gathering

❏   Asked one question at a time and avoided jargon
❏   Used both open-ended and directed questions
❏   Clarified and summarized appropriately
❏   Ensured that patient understood questions asked
❏   Ensured that patient's concerns were addressed and closed interview

*See Global Process Evaluation Criteria (page 10) for a complete evaluation of the interview process.

POST-ENCOUNTER PROBES

Q1. Give five instances when a physician should be concerned about the level of competency of a patient.

i.   When there is evidence of confusion and irrational thinking
ii.   When a patient has short- and/or long-term memory deficits
iii.   If alertness or decisions made fluctuate rapidly
iv.   If the burden of suffering is so great as to impair decision making
v.   If the person is intoxicated with drugs, alcohol, or underlying medical condition

Q2. Provide examples of patients who may be referred for competency assessments by mistake.

i.   Patients of advanced age
ii.   Poorly educated patients
iii.   Physically disabled patients
iv.   Patients who have difficulty in verbal communication (e.g., dysarthric or cannot speak doctor's language)
v.   Patients with different cultural or religious background
vi.   Patients who refuse treatment
vii.   Patients with odd or idiosyncratic beliefs
viii.   Patients with a psychiatric illness

Q3. When would a patient be required to stay in hospital for an involuntary assessment?

i.   The patient has attempted or threatened self-harm.
ii.   The patient has attempted or threatened harm to another.
iii.   The patient has demonstrated a lack of competence in self-care.
iv.   The patient has a mental disorder likely to result in serious bodily harm or harm to others or that will seriously impair the person physically.

Evaluation: Assessment for Elder Abuse

INSTRUCTIONS FOR CANDIDATE

You are the new physician hired to work in a regional geriatrics program. The social worker on your team has raised concerns after a recent home assessment for Elsie Zimmerman, a 76-year-old senior citizen. She now lives with her daughter and son-in-law's family. The social worker was concerned about malnourishment and bruising on her cheek. Perform a directed history and physical examination.

EVALUATION CRITERIA

I. Screens
- ❏ Inquires about Life at Home
- ❏ Inquires about Recent Life Events
- ❏ Inquires about Need for Assistance and Safety

II. Inquiries about Risk Factors for Elder Abuse

i. Abused Victim
- ❏ Psychiatric or Cognitive Problems
- ❏ Alcohol/Substance Abuse

ii. Family of Senior
- ❏ Difficult Family Relationships
- ❏ Past Abuse in Family
- ❏ Ethnocultural Values toward Seniors

iii. Suspected Abuser
- ❏ Psychiatric or Cognitive Problems
- ❏ Alcohol/Substance Abuse
- ❏ Stress Related to Providing Elder Care
- ❏ Poor Respite from Caregiver Role
- ❏ Poor Attitude toward Elder or Caregiver Role
- ❏ Poor Understanding of or Ability to Meet Elder's Needs

III. Positive Indicators

i. Comments on Behaviour During Interview
- ❏ (anxious, agitated, evasive, withdrawn, depressed)

ii. Comments on Behaviour with Caregiver
- ❏ (fearful of caregiver)

iii. Comments on Personal Conduct/Habits
- ❏ Abrupt Change in Social Habits

- ❏ Abrupt Change in Living Arrangements
- ❏ Abrupt Financial Concerns (e.g., inability to pay bills, will changes)
- ❏ Abrupt Cancellations in Medical Appointments

IV. Abusive Event(s)
- ❏ Type of Abuse(s)
- ❏ First Onset and Frequency of Occurrences
- ❏ Consequences of Abuse(s)
- ❏ Perceived Trigger(s) or Cause(s)
- ❏ Actions of Victim During Abuse(s)
- ❏ Actions of Victim to Prevent Abuse(s)

V. Screens for Physical Stigmata of Abuse
i. General Observations
- ❏ Poor Personal Hygiene
- ❏ Dehydration (decr. JVP, BP, incr. HR, etc.)
- ❏ Malnourishment (weight loss, muscle wasting, etc.)

ii. Inspection of Skin
- ❏ Injuries (bruising, lacerations in variable stages of healing) on:
- ❏   Face and Neck
- ❏   Arms and Wrists
- ❏   Inner Thighs and Ankles
- ❏ Skin Ulcerations

iii. Inspection of GU System
- ❏ Genital Rash
- ❏ Genital Bleeding/Bruising
- ❏ Genital Discharge

VI. Process Evaluation*

i. Interpersonal Skills
- ❏ Was aware of patient's nonverbal cues and emotional content
- ❏ Used reflection, checked accuracy of understanding

ii. Information Gathering
- ❏ Asked one question at a time and avoided jargon
- ❏ Used both open-ended and directed questions
- ❏ Clarified and summarized appropriately
- ❏ Ensured that patient understood questions asked
- ❏ Ensured that patient's concerns were addressed and closed interview

*See Global Process Evaluation Criteria (page 10) for a complete evaluation of the interview process.

POST-ENCOUNTER PROBES

Q1. Identify four reasons why abused seniors fail to speak out about their mistreatment.

Fear, shame, lack of knowledge or recognition of abuse, anxiety about the consequences of reporting abuse, belief that it is a private family matter, fear of abandonment, fear of retaliation or rationalization ("I deserve this because I'm too much trouble.")

Q2. Describe the kinds of elder abuse.

Physical Abuse — shaking, pushing, slapping, beating, confinement, forced feeding

Sexual Abuse — forced or unwanted sexual acts such as kissing, fondling, intercourse

Psychological Abuse — threatening, humiliation, name-calling, forced isolation, or unwanted choices

Financial Abuse — theft of money or possessions, forgery, forced control of money such as pension cheques, fraud, extortion, abuse of power of attorney

Neglect — abandonment, failure to provide adequate food, shelter, medical care, clothing, physical aids, or items for personal hygiene and safety

Q3. Clues to elder abuse may be most apparent in an elder's home. If you were visiting one of your senior patients at home, what things in the environment might suggest abuse?

Poor living conditions out of keeping with potential resources, unkempt or dangerous environment, separation from others in home, evidence of locks or restraints, restricted access to telephone, inappropriate/inadequate/soiled clothing, lack of food, lack of medications, and lack of medical or functional devices (eyeglasses, hearing aids, walkers, wheelchairs, etc.)

Part VI

Abbreviations

AAA	Abdominal Aortic Aneurysm	Incr.	Increased
ADLs	Activities of Daily Living	IUD	Intra-Uterine Device
AntiHBs	Antibodies against Hepatitis B Surface Antigen	JVP	Jugular Venous Pressure
		L	Left
		LH	Luteinizing Hormone
ASD	Atrial Septal Defect	LLD	Left Lateral Decubitus
AXR	Abdominal X-Ray	LOC	Level of Consciousness
BP	Blood Pressure	LVH	Left Ventricular Hypertrophy
BPH	Benign Prostatic Hyperplasia	MCP	Metacarpal–Phalangeal
BUN	Blood Urea Nitrogen	MSK	Musculoskeletal
C&S	Culture and Sensitivities	MSS	Maternal Serum Screen
CAD	Coronary Artery Disease	MTP	Metatarsal–Phalangeal
CBC	Complete Blood Count	NYHA	New York Heart Association
CGD	Congenital Growth Delay	OCP	Oral Contraceptive Pill
CHF	Congestive Heart Failure	OTC	Over the Counter
CN	Cranial Nerve	Pap	Papanicolaou's Cervical Smear
CVS	Chronic Villous Sampling		
COPD	Chronic Obstructive Pulmonary Disease	PCOD	Polycystic Ovarian Disease
Cr	Creatinine	PE	Physical Examination
CT	Computer Tomography	PID	Pelvic Inflammatory Disease
CVA	Cerebral Vascular Accident	PIP	Proximal Interphalangeal Joint
CVD	Coronary Vascular Disease	PMI	Point of Maximal Impulse
CVS	Chronic Villous Sampling	PR	Pulse Rate
CXR	Chest X-Ray	Pt	Patient
DDx	Differential Diagnosis	PVD	Peripheral Vascular Disease
Decr.	Decreased		
DIP	Distal Interphalangeal Joint	R	Right
		RBC	Red Blood Cells
DM	Diabetes Mellitus	RF	Risk Factors
DRE	Digital Rectal Exam	RML	Right Middle Lobe
Dx	Diagnosis	ROM	Range of Motion
EEG	Electroencephalogram	RR	Respiration Rate
EKG	Electrocardiogram	Rx	Treatment
EtOH	Ethanol Alcohol	SOB	Shortness of Breath
FHx	Family History	T3	Thyroxine
FSH	Follicular Stimulating Hormone	TB	Tuberculosis
		TIA	Transient Ischemic Attack
FSS	Familial Short Stature	TSH	Thyroid-Stimulating Hormone
FTT	Failure to Thrive		
GI	Gastrointestinal	Tx	Treatment
GU	Genitourinary	U/S	Ultrasound
HbsAg	Hepatitis B Surface Antigen	UTI	Urinary Tract Infection
		VDRL	Venereal Disease Reference Laboratory
HIV	Human Immunodeficiency Virus		
		VS	Vital Signs
Hx	History	WBC	White Blood Cells
IADLs	Instrumental Activities of Daily Living	y	Year(s)

Part VII

References

II. SCENARIOS FOR DIRECTED HISTORIES

Amenorrhea

1. Andreoli TE, Carpenter CCJ, Griggs RC, Loscalzo JC. *Cecil Essentials of Medicine*. 5th ed. New York: W.B. Saunders Company; 2001:612–613.
2. Rouse T, Tang G, Torgerson C, Van Spall H. *Essentials of Clinical Examination Handbook*. 3rd ed. Toronto: The Medical Society, Faculty of Medicine, University of Toronto; 2000:115–116.
3. Yue J, Ahuja G. *Toronto Notes—MCCQE 2001 Review Notes*. 17th ed. Toronto: The Medical Society, Faculty of Medicine, University of Toronto; 2001:GY10–11.

Anemia

1. Andreoli TE, Carpenter CCJ, Griggs RC, Loscalzo JC. *Cecil Essentials of Medicine*. 5th ed. New York: W.B. Saunders Company; 2001:419–430.
2. Yue J, Ahuja G. *Toronto Notes—MCCQE 2001 Review Notes*. 17th ed. Toronto: The Medical Society, Faculty of Medicine, University of Toronto; 2001:H3.

Benign Prostatic Hyperplasia (BPH)

1. Andreoli TE, Carpenter CCJ, Griggs RC, Loscalzo JC. *Cecil Essentials of Medicine*. 5th ed. New York: W.B. Saunders Company; 2001:1008–1009.
2. Rouse T, Tang G, Torgerson C, Van Spall H. *Essentials of Clinical Examination Handbook*. 3rd ed. Toronto: The Medical Society, Faculty of Medicine, University of Toronto; 2000:156.
3. Yue J, Ahuja G. *Toronto Notes—MCCQE 2001 Review Notes*. 17th ed. Toronto: The Medical Society, Faculty of Medicine, University of Toronto; 2001:U18–19.

Diabetes

1. Andreoli TE, Carpenter CCJ, Griggs RC, Loscalzo JC. *Cecil Essentials of Medicine*. 5th ed. New York: W.B. Saunders Company; 2001:583–598.
2. CMA. 1998 clinical practice guidelines for the management of diabetes in Canada. *Supplement to Can Med Assoc J* 1998;159(8 Suppl).
3. Institute for Clinical Evaluative Sciences. A new script: oral hypoglycemic therapy in type 2 diabetes. *Informed 2002*; 8(3):1–4.
4. Yue J, Ahuja G. *Toronto Notes—MCCQE 2001 Review Notes*. 17th ed. Toronto: The Medical Society, Faculty of Medicine, University of Toronto; 2001:E2–E8.

Diarrhea

1. Andreoli TE, Carpenter CCJ, Griggs RC, Loscalzo JC. *Cecil Essentials of Medicine*. 5th ed. New York: W.B. Saunders Company; 2001:316–320.
2. Yue J, Ahuja G. *Toronto Notes—MCCQE 2001 Review Notes*. 17th ed. Toronto: The Medical Society, Faculty of Medicine, University of Toronto; 2001:G10–16.

Elderly

1. Andreoli TE, Carpenter CCJ, Griggs RC, Loscalzo JC. *Cecil Essentials of Medicine*. 5th ed. New York: W.B. Saunders Company; 2001:1006–1010.
2. Rouse T, Tang G, Torgerson C, Van Spall H. *Essentials of Clinical Examination Handbook*. 3rd ed. Toronto: The Medical Society, Faculty of Medicine, University of Toronto; 2000:223–234.
3. Yue J, Ahuja G. *Toronto Notes—MCCQE 2001 Review Notes*. 17th ed. Toronto: The Medical Society, Faculty of Medicine, University of Toronto; 2001:GM4–5.

Erectile Dysfunction

1. Efficacy and safety of sildenafil citrate for the treatment of erectile dysfunction in men with cardiovascular disease. *Internatl J Clin Pract* 2001;55(3):171–176.

2. NIH Consensus Development Panel on Impotence. Impotence. *JAMA* 1993; 270(1):83–90.

3. Rouse T, Tang G, Torgerson C, Van Spall H. *Essentials of Clinical Examination Handbook*. 3rd ed. Toronto: The Medical Society, Faculty of Medicine, University of Toronto; 2000:157.

Failure to Thrive

1. Cheng A, Jacobson S. Failure to thrive: approach to diagnosis and management. *U Toronto Med J* 1999;75(1):4–9.

2. Rouse T, Tang G, Torgerson C, Van Spall H. *Essentials of Clinical Examination Handbook*. 3rd ed. Toronto: The Medical Society, Faculty of Medicine, University of Toronto; 2000:201–206.

3. Yue J, Ahuja G. *Toronto Notes—MCCQE 2001 Review Notes*. 17th ed. Toronto: The Medical Society, Faculty of Medicine, University of Toronto; 2001:P10–11.

Fever

1. Andreoli TE, Carpenter CCJ, Griggs RC, Loscalzo JC. *Cecil Essentials of Medicine*. 5th ed. New York: W.B. Saunders Company; 2001:750–764.

2. Yue J, Ahuja G. *Toronto Notes—MCCQE 2001 Review Notes*. 17th ed. Toronto: The Medical Society, Faculty of Medicine, University of Toronto; 2001:P48.

Gay and Lesbian Health Issues

1. Davis, V. SOGC clinical practice guidelines. Lesbian health guidelines. *J Soc Obstet Gynaecol Can* 2000;22(3):202–205.

2. *Gay & Lesbian Health Issues*. (Unpublished.) Toronto: University of Toronto, 2000.

Headache

1. Andreoli TE, Carpenter CCJ, Griggs RC, Loscalzo JC. *Cecil Essentials of Medicine*. 5th ed. New York: W.B. Saunders Company; 2001:909–912.

2. Smetana GW, Shmerling RH. Does this patient have temporal arteritis? *JAMA* 2002;287:92–101.

3. William EM, Pryse-Phillips MD, et al. Guidelines for the diagnosis and management of migraine in clinical practice. 1991. *Can Med Assoc J* 1991;56(9): 1273–1287.

4. Yue J, Ahuja G. *Toronto Notes—MCCQE 2001 Review Notes*. 17th ed. Toronto: The Medical Society, Faculty of Medicine, University of Toronto; 2001:FM 23–25.

HIV

1. Andreoli TE, Carpenter CCJ, Griggs RC, Loscalzo JC. *Cecil Essentials of Medicine*. 5th ed. New York: W.B. Saunders Company; 2001:847–850.

2. Rouse T, Tang G, Torgerson C, Van Spall H. *Essentials of Clinical Examination Handbook*. 3rd ed. Toronto: The Medical Society, Faculty of Medicine, University of Toronto; 2000:24–25.

3. Yue J, Ahuja G. *Toronto Notes—MCCQE 2001 Review Notes*. 17th ed. Toronto: The Medical Society, Faculty of Medicine, University of Toronto; 2001:ID52–56.

Hypertension (Management)

1. Andreoli TE, Carpenter CCJ, Griggs RC, Loscalzo JC. *Cecil Essentials of Medicine*. 5th ed. New York: W.B. Saunders Company; 2001:158–159.

2. CMA. 1999 Canadian recommendations for the management of hypertension including case-based applications of the recommendations. *Can Med Assoc J* 1999;161(12 Suppl):S1–S21.

3. Gray J. *Therapeutic Choices*. 3rd ed. Ottawa: Canadian Pharmacists Association; 2000:188.

4. Yue J, Ahuja G. *Toronto Notes—MCCQE 2001 Review Notes*. 17th ed. Toronto: The Medical Society, Faculty of Medicine, University of Toronto; 2001:FM11–14.

Insomnia

1. Andreoli TE, Carpenter CCJ, Griggs RC, Loscalzo JC. *Cecil Essentials of Medicine*. 5th ed. New York: W.B. Saunders Company; 2001:890.

2. Institute for Clinical Evaluative Sciences. Are you getting enough … zzzz? *Informed* 2001;7(3):1–4.

3. Shapiro C, Fleming J, Flanigan M, et al. *Sleep Solutions Manual*. 1st ed. Pointe Claire: Kommunicom Publications; 1995:7–12, 34–40.

Menorrhagia

1. Andreoli TE, Carpenter CCJ, Griggs RC, Loscalzo JC. *Cecil Essentials of Medicine*. 5th ed. New York: W.B. Saunders Company; 2001:613–616.

2. SOGC. Guidelines for the management of abnormal uterine bleeding. *J Soc Obstet Gynaecol Can* 2001;23(8):704–709.

3. Yue J, Ahuja G. *Toronto Notes—MCCQE 2001 Review Notes*. 17th ed. Toronto: The Medical Society, Faculty of Medicine, University of Toronto; 2001:GY11–13.

Nausea and Vomiting

1. Andreoli TE, Carpenter CCJ, Griggs RC, Loscalzo JC. *Cecil Essentials of Medicine*. 5th ed. New York: W.B. Saunders Company; 2001:307, 519–520

2. Yue J, Ahuja G. *Toronto Notes—MCCQE 2001 Review Notes*. 17th ed. Toronto: The Medical Society, Faculty of Medicine, University of Toronto; 2001:P31–33, G1–43.

Obstructed Bowel

1. Lawrence PF. *Essentials of General Surgery*. 3rd ed. Philadelphia: Lippincott Williams & Wilkins; 2000:255–259.

2. Yue J, Ahuja G. *Toronto Notes—MCCQE 2001 Review Notes*. 17th ed. Toronto: The Medical Society, Faculty of Medicine, University of Toronto; 2001:GS15–16.

Oliguria

1. Andreoli TE, Carpenter CCJ, Griggs RC, Loscalzo JC. *Cecil Essentials of Medicine*. 5th ed. New York: W.B. Saunders Company; 2001:284, 286–287, 294.

2. Yue J, Ahuja G. *Toronto Notes—MCCQE 2001 Review Notes*. 17th ed. Toronto: The Medical Society, Faculty of Medicine, University of Toronto; 2001:NP7, 17–20.

Oral Contraception
1. Rouse T, Tang G, Torgerson C, Van Spall H. *Essentials of Clinical Examination Handbook*. 3rd ed. Toronto: The Medical Society, Faculty of Medicine, University of Toronto; 2000:24–25.
2. Yue J, Ahuja G. *Toronto Notes—MCCQE 2001 Review Notes*. 17th ed. Toronto: The Medical Society, Faculty of Medicine, University of Toronto; 2001:GY3, GY19.

Otitis Media
1. Andreoli TE, Carpenter CCJ, Griggs RC, Loscalzo JC. *Cecil Essentials of Medicine*. 5th ed. New York: W.B. Saunders Company; 2001:782.
2. Institute for Clinical Evaluative Sciences. 'Ear today. Gone tomorrow? Controversies in the management of otitis media in children. *Informed* 2000;7(1):1–5.
3. Yue J, Ahuja G. *Toronto Notes—MCCQE 2001 Review Notes*. 17th ed. Toronto: The Medical Society, Faculty of Medicine, University of Toronto; 2001:OT26–28.

Overdose
1. Yue J, Ahuja G. *Toronto Notes—MCCQE 2001 Review Notes*. 17th ed. Toronto: The Medical Society, Faculty of Medicine, University of Toronto; 2001:PS25–26.

Palpitations (Heart)
1. Andreoli TE, Carpenter CCJ, Griggs RC, Loscalzo JC. *Cecil Essentials of Medicine*. 5th ed. New York: W.B. Saunders Company; 2001:100–126.
2. Yue J, Ahuja G. *Toronto Notes—MCCQE 2001 Review Notes*. 17th ed. Toronto: The Medical Society, Faculty of Medicine, University of Toronto; 2001:C13–20.

Physical Abuse
1. Baldwin L. Violence against women: what can physicians do? *Can J Cont Med Educ* July 1995:19–25.
2. Rouse T, Tang G, Torgerson C, Van Spall H. *Essentials of Clinical Examination Handbook*. 3rd ed. Toronto: The Medical Society, Faculty of Medicine, University of Toronto; 2000:27–29.

Postoperative Fever
1. Lawrence PF. *Essentials of General Surgery*. 3rd ed. Philadelphia: Lippincott Williams & Wilkins; 2000.
2. Sullivan P. *Anaesthesia for Medical Students*. 2nd ed. Ottawa: Department of Anesthesia, Ottawa Civic Hospital, 1999; 194–206.
3. Yue J, Ahuja G. *Toronto Notes—MCCQE 2001 Review Notes*. 17th ed. Toronto: The Medical Society, Faculty of Medicine, University of Toronto; 2001:GS2–5.

Preoperative Patient
1. *Handbook of Clinical Anesthesia*. 2nd ed. New York: J.B. Lippincott Company; 1993:3–15.
2. Lawrence PF. *Essentials of General Surgery*. 3rd ed. Philadelphia: Lippincott Williams & Wilkins; 2000.
3. Sullivan P. *Anaesthesia for Medical Students*. 2nd ed. Ottawa: Department of Anesthesia, Ottawa Civic Hospital; 1999:9–26.

Renal Colic

1. Andreoli TE, Carpenter CCJ, Griggs RC, Loscalzo JC. *Cecil Essentials of Medicine*. 5th ed. New York: W.B. Saunders Company; 2001:272–277.

2. Rouse T, Tang G, Torgerson C, Van Spall H. *Essentials of Clinical Examination Handbook*. 3rd ed. Toronto: The Medical Society, Faculty of Medicine, University of Toronto; 2000:165.

3. Yue J, Ahuja G. *Toronto Notes—MCCQE 2001 Review Notes*. 17th ed. Toronto: The Medical Society, Faculty of Medicine, University of Toronto; 2001:U2–6.

Seizures

1. Andreoli TE, Carpenter CCJ, Griggs RC, Loscalzo JC. Cecil *Essentials of Medicine*. 5th ed. New York: W.B. Saunders Company; 2001:956–964.

2. Rouse T, Tang G, Torgerson C, Van Spall H. *Essentials of Clinical Examination Handbook*. 3rd ed. Toronto: The Medical Society, Faculty of Medicine, University of Toronto; 2000:131–154.

3. Yue J, Ahuja G. *Toronto Notes—MCCQE 2001 Review Notes*. 17th ed. Toronto: The Medical Society, Faculty of Medicine, University of Toronto; 2001:N8–13.

Sexual Abuse

1. Baldwin L. Violence against women: what can physicians do? *Can J Cont Med Educ* July 1995:19–25.

2. Finkel KC. Sexual abuse and incest. *Can Fam Physician* 1994;40:935–944.

3. Rouse T, Tang G, Torgerson C, Van Spall H. *Essentials of Clinical Examination Handbook*. 3rd ed. Toronto: The Medical Society, Faculty of Medicine, University of Toronto; 2000:27–29.

Sexually Transmitted Diseases

1. Andreoli TE, Carpenter CCJ, Griggs RC, Loscalzo JC. Cecil *Essentials of Medicine*. 5th ed. New York: W.B. Saunders Company; 2001:832–840.

2. Rouse T, Tang G, Torgerson C, Van Spall H. *Essentials of Clinical Examination Handbook*. 3rd ed. Toronto: The Medical Society, Faculty of Medicine, University of Toronto; 2000:24–25, 179–180.

3. Yue J, Ahuja G. *Toronto Notes—MCCQE 2001 Review Notes*. 17th ed. Toronto: The Medical Society, Faculty of Medicine, University of Toronto; 2001:FM26, GY26–30.

Urinary Tract Infection

1. Siberry GK, Iannone R. *The Harriet Lane Handbook*. 15th ed. Toronto: Mosby; 2000.

2. Dipchang AI. *The HSC Handbook of Pediatrics*. 9th ed. Toronto: Mosby, 1997; 62–466.

3. Yue J, Ahuja G. *Toronto Notes—MCCQE 2001 Review Notes*. 17th ed. Toronto: The Medical Society, Faculty of Medicine, University of Toronto; 2001:80–81.

Well Baby

1. Bates B, Bickley LS, Hoekelman RA. *A Guide to Physical Examination and History Taking*. 6th ed. Philadelphia: J.B. Lippincott Company; 1995:555–560.

2. Rouse T, Tang G, Torgerson C, Van Spall H. *Essentials of Clinical Examination Handbook*. 3rd ed. Toronto: The Medical Society, Faculty of Medicine, University of Toronto; 2000:201–205.

3. Yue J, Ahuja G. *Toronto Notes—MCCQE 2001 Review Notes*. 17th ed. Toronto: The Medical Society, Faculty of Medicine, University of Toronto; 2001:P1–P10.

III. SCENARIOS FOR DIRECTED HISTORIES AND PHYSICAL EXAMINATIONS

Acute Abdomen

1. Andreoli TE, Carpenter CCJ, Griggs RC, Loscalzo JC. *Cecil Essentials of Medicine*. 5th ed. New York: W.B. Saunders Company; 2001:305.
2. Bates B, Bickley LS, Hoekelman RA. *A Guide to Physical Examination and History Taking*. 6th ed. Philadelphia: J.B. Lippincott Company; 1995:335–360.
3. Lawrence PF. *Essentials of General Surgery*. 3rd ed. Philadelphia: Lippincott Williams & Wilkins; 2000:130.
4. Rouse T, Tang G, Torgerson C, Van Spall H. *Essentials of Clinical Examination Handbook*. 3rd ed. Toronto: The Medical Society, Faculty of Medicine, University of Toronto; 2000:99–108.
5. Yue J, Ahuja G. *Toronto Notes—MCCQE 2001 Review Notes*. 17th ed. Toronto: The Medical Society, Faculty of Medicine, University of Toronto; 2001:GS6–8.

Alcoholism

1. Andreoli TE, Carpenter CCJ, Griggs RC, Loscalzo JC. *Cecil Essentials of Medicine*. 5th ed. New York: W.B. Saunders Company; 2001:1014–1018.
2. Kitchens J. Does this patient have an alcohol problem? *JAMA* 1994;272:1782–1787.
3. Rouse T, Tang G, Torgerson C, Van Spall H. *Essentials of Clinical Examination Handbook*. 3rd ed. Toronto: The Medical Society, Faculty of Medicine, University of Toronto; 2000:25–26.
4. Yue J, Ahuja G. *Toronto Notes—MCCQE 2001 Review Notes*. 17th ed. Toronto: The Medical Society, Faculty of Medicine, University of Toronto; 2001:FM5–6, G33.

Asthma

1. Boulet L-P, Becker A, Berube D, Beveridge R, Ernst P. Summary of recommendations from the Canadian asthma consensus report, 1999. *Can Med Assoc J* 1999;161(11):s1–s12.
2. Chawla A, Somani R. *Essentials of Clinical Examination Handbook*. 2nd ed. Toronto: The Medical Society, Faculty of Medicine, University of Toronto; 2000:23–30.
3. Dipchang AI. *The HSC Handbook of Pediatrics*. 9th ed. Toronto: Mosby; 1997:462–466.

Back Pain

1. Bates B, Bickley LS, Hoekelman RA. *A Guide to Physical Examination and History Taking*. 6th ed. Philadelphia: J.B. Lippincott Company; 1995:477–479.
2. Biogos S, Bowyer O, Braen G, et al. *Acute Low Back Problems in Adults*. Clinical Practice Guideline, Quick Reference Guide Number 14. Rockville, MD: US Department of Health and Human Services, Public Health Service, Agency for Health Care Policy and Research, AHCPR Pub. No. 95-0643. December 1994.

3. Rouse T, Tang G, Torgerson C, Van Spall H. *Essentials of Clinical Examination Handbook*. 3rd ed. Toronto: The Medical Society, Faculty of Medicine, University of Toronto; 2000:121–124.

4. Yue J, Ahuja G. *Toronto Notes—MCCQE 2001 Review Notes*. 17th ed. Toronto: The Medical Society, Faculty of Medicine, University of Toronto; 2001:FM32.

Breast Lump

1. Bates B, Bickley LS, Hoekelman RA. *A Guide to Physical Examination and History Taking*. 6th ed. Philadelphia: J.B. Lippincott Company; 1995:320–329.

2. Lawrence PF. *Essentials of General Surgery*. 3rd ed. Philadelphia: Lippincott Williams & Wilkins; 2000:368–385.

3. Rouse T, Tang G, Torgerson C, Van Spall H. *Essentials of Clinical Examination Handbook*. 3rd ed. Toronto: The Medical Society, Faculty of Medicine, University of Toronto; 2000:167–172.

4. Yue J, Ahuja G. *Toronto Notes—MCCQE 2001 Review Notes*. 17th ed. Toronto: The Medical Society, Faculty of Medicine, University of Toronto; 2001:GS41–45.

Chest Pain

1. Andreoli TE, Carpenter CCJ, Griggs RC, Loscalzo JC. *Cecil Essentials of Medicine*. 5th ed. New York: W.B. Saunders Company; 2001:79–99.

2. Bates B, Bickley LS, Hoekelman RA. *A Guide to Physical Examination and History Taking*. 6th ed. Philadelphia: J.B. Lippincott Company; 1995:285–299.

3. New Advances in the management of acute coronary syndromes: matching treatment to risk. *Can Med Assoc J* 2001; 164(9):1309–1316.

4. Rouse T, Tang G, Torgerson C, Van Spall H. *Essentials of Clinical Examination Handbook*. 3rd ed. Toronto: The Medical Society, Faculty of Medicine, University of Toronto; 2000:65–75.

5. Yue J, Ahuja G. *Toronto Notes—MCCQE 2001 Review Notes*. 17th ed. Toronto: The Medical Society, Faculty of Medicine, University of Toronto; 2001:C8–10.

Congestive Heart Failure

1. Andreoli TE, Carpenter CCJ, Griggs RC, Loscalzo JC. *Cecil Essentials of Medicine*. 5th ed. New York: W.B. Saunders Company; 2001:56–62.

2. The 2001 Canadian Cardiovascular Society consensus guideline update for the management and prevention of heart failure. *Canadian Journal of Cardiology* 17 (Suppl E):1E –24E

3. Yue J, Ahuja G. *Toronto Notes—MCCQE 2001 Review Notes*. 17th ed. Toronto: The Medical Society, Faculty of Medicine, University of Toronto; 2001:C31–35.

Cough

1. Andreoli TE, Carpenter CCJ, Griggs RC, Loscalzo JC. *Cecil Essentials of Medicine*. 5th ed. New York: W.B. Saunders Company; 2001:788–797.

2. Fine MJ, Auble TE, Yealy DM, et al. 1997. A prediction rule to identify low-risk patients with community-acquired pneumonia. *New Engl J Med* 1997; 336(4):243–250.

3. Rouse T, Tang G, Torgerson C, Van Spall H. *Essentials of Clinical Examination Handbook*. 3rd ed. Toronto: The Medical Society, Faculty of Medicine, University of Toronto; 2000:56–58.

4. Yue J, Ahuja G. *Toronto Notes—MCCQE 2001 Review Notes*. 17th ed. Toronto: The Medical Society, Faculty of Medicine, University of Toronto; 2001:R31–34.

Craniofacial Trauma
1. Yue J, Ahuja G. *Toronto Notes—MCCQE 2001 Review Notes*. 17th ed. Toronto: The Medical Society, Faculty of Medicine, University of Toronto; 2001:PL19.

Dementia
1. Folstein MF, Folstein SE, McHugh PR. "Mini-mental state": a practical method of grading the cognitive state of patients for the clinician. *J Psychiatric Res* 1975;12:189–198.
2. Management of dementing disorders. Conclusions from the Canadian Consensus Conference on Dementia. *Supplement to Can Med Assoc J* 1999; 160.
3. Yue J, Ahuja G. *Toronto Notes—MCCQE 2001 Review Notes*. 17th ed. Toronto: The Medical Society, Faculty of Medicine, University of Toronto; 2001:PS17–18.

Eating Disorders
1. Andreoli TE, Carpenter CCJ, Griggs RC, Loscalzo JC. *Cecil Essentials of Medicine*. 5th ed. New York: W.B. Saunders Company; 2001:519–521.
2. Rouse T, Tang G, Torgerson C, Van Spall H. *Essentials of Clinical Examination Handbook*. 3rd ed. Toronto: The Medical Society, Faculty of Medicine, University of Toronto; 2000:247.
3. Yue J, Ahuja G. *Toronto Notes—MCCQE 2001 Review Notes*. 17th ed. Toronto: The Medical Society, Faculty of Medicine, University of Toronto; 2001:P33–34.

Hand Trauma
1. Bates B, Bickley LS, Hoekelman RA. *A Guide to Physical Examination and History Taking*. 6th ed. Philadelphia: J.B. Lippincott Company; 1995:450–451
2. Rouse T, Tang G, Torgerson C, Van Spall H. *Essentials of Clinical Examination Handbook*. 3rd ed. Toronto: The Medical Society, Faculty of Medicine, University of Toronto; 2000:119–121.
3. Yue J, Ahuja G. *Toronto Notes—MCCQE 2001 Review Notes*. 17th ed. Toronto: The Medical Society, Faculty of Medicine, University of Toronto; 2001:PL8–10.

Meningitis
1. Andreoli TE, Carpenter CCJ, Griggs RC, Loscalzo JC. *Cecil Essentials of Medicine*. 5th ed. New York: W.B. Saunders Company; 2001:772–777.
2. Rouse T, Tang G, Torgerson C, Van Spall H. *Essentials of Clinical Examination Handbook*. 3rd ed. Toronto: The Medical Society, Faculty of Medicine, University of Toronto; 2000:249–250.
3. Yue J, Ahuja G. *Toronto Notes—MCCQE 2001 Review Notes*. 17th ed. Toronto: The Medical Society, Faculty of Medicine, University of Toronto; 2001:N57–N58.

Obesity
1. Andreoli TE, Carpenter CCJ, Griggs RC, Loscalzo JC. *Cecil Essentials of Medicine*. 5th ed. New York: W.B. Saunders Company; 2001:517–518.
2. Douketis JD, John W, et al. Periodic health examination, 1999 update: 1. detection, prevention and treatment of obesity. *Can Med Assoc J* 1999;160:513–525.

3. Yue J, Ahuja G. *Toronto Notes—MCCQE 2001 Review Notes*. 17th ed. Toronto: The Medical Society, Faculty of Medicine, University of Toronto; 2001:E13–14.

Peripheral Vascular Disease
1. Bates B, Bickley LS, Hoekelman RA. *A Guide to Physical Examination and History Taking*. 6th ed. Philadelphia: J.B. Lippincott Company; 1995:433–447.
2. Rouse T, Tang G, Torgerson C, Van Spall H. *Essentials of Clinical Examination Handbook*. 3rd ed. Toronto: The Medical Society, Faculty of Medicine, University of Toronto; 2000:84–88.
3. Yue J, Ahuja G. *Toronto Notes—MCCQE 2001 Review Notes*. 17th ed. Toronto: The Medical Society, Faculty of Medicine, University of Toronto; 2001:GS46–50.

Rheumatoid Arthritis
1. Bates B, Bickley LS, Hoekelman RA. *A Guide to Physical Examination and History Taking*. 6th ed. Philadelphia: J.B. Lippincott Company; 1995:464–490.
2. Rouse T, Tang G, Torgerson C, Van Spall H. *Essentials of Clinical Examination Handbook*. 3rd ed. Toronto: The Medical Society, Faculty of Medicine, University of Toronto; 2000:113–130.
3. Yue J, Ahuja G. *Toronto Notes—MCCQE 2001 Review Notes*. 17th ed. Toronto: The Medical Society, Faculty of Medicine, University of Toronto; 2001:RH9–11.

Stroke
1. Findlay JM, Tucker WS, Ferguson GG, et al. Guidelines for the use of carotid endarterectomy: current recommendations from the Canadian Neurosurgical Society. *Can Med Assoc J* 1997;157(6):653.
2. Moira K, Kapral MK, Silver FL. Preventive health care, 1999 update: 2. Echocardiography for the detection of a cardiac source of embolus in patients with stroke. *Can Med Assoc J* 1999;161(8):989–996.
3. Rouse T, Tang G, Torgerson C, Van Spall H. *Essentials of Clinical Examination Handbook*. 3rd ed. Toronto: The Medical Society, Faculty of Medicine, University of Toronto; 2000:133–145.

Thyroid
1. Bates B, Bickley LS, Hoekelman RA. *A Guide to Physical Examination and History Taking*. 6th ed. Philadelphia: J.B. Lippincott Company; 1995:188–190.
2. Rouse T, Tang G, Torgerson C, Van Spall H. *Essentials of Clinical Examination Handbook*. 3rd ed. Toronto: The Medical Society, Faculty of Medicine, University of Toronto; 2000:36–41.
3. Yue J, Ahuja G. *Toronto Notes—MCCQE 2001 Review Notes*. 17th ed. Toronto: The Medical Society, Faculty of Medicine, University of Toronto; 2001:E19–E24.

Trauma (Primary Survey)
1. Cass D, Fulton L, Mazurik L, Rutledge T, Schwartz B, Yaphe J. *Introduction to Emergency Medicine*. 4th ed. Toronto: Department of Emergency Medicine, University of Toronto; 1999: 23–38, 229–243.
2. Weissleder R, Rieumont MJ, Wittenberg J. *Primer of Diagnostic Imaging*. 2nd ed. Toronto: Mosby; 1997: 346–347

3. Yue J, Ahuja G. *Toronto Notes—MCCQE 2001 Review Notes*. 17th ed. Toronto: The Medical Society, Faculty of Medicine, University of Toronto; 2001: ER2–ER26.

Trauma (Secondary Survey)

1. Cass D, Fulton L, Mazurik L, Rutledge T, Schwartz B, Yaphe J. *Introduction to Emergency Medicine*. 4th ed. Toronto: Department of Emergency Medicine, University of Toronto; 1999: 23–38, 229–243.

2. Weissleder R, Rieumont MJ, Wittenberg J. *Primer of Diagnostic Imaging*. 2nd ed. Toronto: Mosby; 1997: 346–347.

3. Yue J, Ahuja G. *Toronto Notes—MCCQE 2001 Review Notes*. 17th ed. Toronto: The Medical Society, Faculty of Medicine, University of Toronto; 2001: ER2–26.

IV. SCENARIOS FOR PHYSICAL EXAMINATIONS

Coordination

1. Bates B, Bickley LS, Hoekelman RA. *A Guide to Physical Examination and History Taking*. 6th ed. Philadelphia: J.B. Lippincott Company; 1995:518–520.

2. Rouse T, Tang G, Torgerson C, Van Spall H. *Essentials of Clinical Examination Handbook*. 3rd ed. Toronto: The Medical Society, Faculty of Medicine, University of Toronto; 2000:144–145.

3. Yue J, Ahuja G. *Toronto Notes—MCCQE 2001 Review Notes*. 17th ed. Toronto: The Medical Society, Faculty of Medicine, University of Toronto; 2001:N38–39.

Cranial Nerves

1. Bates B, Bickley LS, Hoekelman RA. *A Guide to Physical Examination and History Taking*. 6th ed. Philadelphia: J.B. Lippincott Company; 1995:505–510.

2. Rouse T, Tang G, Torgerson C, Van Spall H. *Essentials of Clinical Examination Handbook*. 3rd ed. Toronto: The Medical Society, Faculty of Medicine, University of Toronto; 2000:133–138

3. Yue J, Ahuja G. *Toronto Notes—MCCQE 2001 Review Notes*. 17th ed. Toronto: The Medical Society, Faculty of Medicine, University of Toronto; 2001:N26–32.

Hip

1. Anderson BC. *Office Orthopedics for Primary Care Diagnosis and Treatment*. 2nd ed. New York: W.B. Saunders Company; 1999:125–137.

2. Bates B, Bickley LS, Hoekelman RA. *A Guide to Physical Examination and History Taking*. 6th ed. Philadelphia: J.B. Lippincott Company; 1995:474–476.

3. Rouse T, Tang G, Torgerson C, Van Spall H. *Essentials of Clinical Examination Handbook*. 3rd ed. Toronto: The Medical Society, Faculty of Medicine, University of Toronto; 2000:113, 125–126.

Hypertension (Complications)

1. CMA. 1999 Canadian recommendations for the management of hypertension including case-based applications of the recommendations. *Can Med Assoc J* 1999;161 (12 Suppl):S1–S21.

2. Swartz MH. *Textbook of Physical Diagnosis: History and Examination*. 4th ed. Philadelphia: W.B. Saunders Company; 2002: 352, 367–372, 399–400.

Knee

1. Ferri FF. *Practical Guide to the Care of the Medical Patient*. 4th ed. Toronto: Mosby; 1998:598–599, 815.
2. Chawla A, Somani R. *Essentials of Clinical Examination Handbook*. 2nd ed. Toronto: The Medical Society, Faculty of Medicine, University of Toronto; 1999:121–134.
3. Yue J, Ahuja G. *Toronto Notes—MCCQE 2001 Review Notes*. 17th ed. Toronto: The Medical Society, Faculty of Medicine, University of Toronto; 2001:OR27–30.

Lymph Nodes

1. Bates B, Bickley LS, Hoekelman RA. *A Guide to Physical Examination and History Taking*. 6th ed. Philadelphia: J.B. Lippincott Company; 1995:187, 430–431.
2. Rouse T, Tang G, Torgerson C, Van Spall H. *Essentials of Clinical Examination Handbook*. 3rd ed. Toronto: The Medical Society, Faculty of Medicine, University of Toronto; 2000:38, 169–170.

Parkinson's Disease

1. Andreoli TE, Carpenter CCJ, Griggs RC, Loscalzo JC. *Cecil Essentials of Medicine*. 5th ed. New York: W.B. Saunders Company; 2001:933–934.
2. Bates B, Bickley LS, Hoekelman RA. *A Guide to Physical Examination and History Taking*. 6th ed. Philadelphia: J.B. Lippincott Company; 1995:510–532.
3. Lindsay KW, Bone I. *Neurology and Neurosurgery Illustrated*. 3rd ed. London: Church Livingstone; 1998:353–354.
4. Rouse T, Tang G, Torgerson C, Van Spall H. *Essentials of Clinical Examination Handbook*. 3rd ed. Toronto: The Medical Society, Faculty of Medicine, University of Toronto; 2000:152.

Pulsus Paradoxus

1. Andreoli TE, Carpenter CCJ, Griggs RC, Loscalzo JC. *Cecil Essentials of Medicine*. 5th ed. New York: W.B. Saunders Company; 2001:134.
2. Rouse T, Tang G, Torgerson C, Van Spall H. *Essentials of Clinical Examination Handbook*. 3rd ed. Toronto: The Medical Society, Faculty of Medicine, University of Toronto; 2000:23.

Shoulder

1. Anderson BC. *Office Orthopedics for Primary Care Diagnosis and Treatment*. 2nd ed. New York: W.B. Saunders Company; 1999:13–45.
2. Bates B, Bickley LS, Hoekelman RA. *A Guide to Physical Examination and History Taking*. 6th ed. Philadelphia: J.B. Lippincott Company; 1995:453–455.
3. Rouse T, Tang G, Torgerson C, Van Spall H. *Essentials of Clinical Examination Handbook*. 3rd ed. Toronto: The Medical Society, Faculty of Medicine, University of Toronto; 2000:113, 115–116.

Volume Status

1. Andreoli TE, Carpenter CCJ, Griggs RC, Loscalzo JC. *Cecil Essentials of Medicine*. 5th ed. New York: W.B. Saunders Company; 2001:239–240.

2. Bates B, Bickley LS, Hoekelman, RA. *A Guide to Physical Examination and History Taking*. 6th ed. Philadelphia: J.B. Lippincott Company; 1995:270–271, 281, 433–438.

3. Rouse T, Tang G, Torgerson C, Van Spall H. *Essentials of Clinical Examination Handbook*. 3rd ed. Toronto: The Medical Society, Faculty of Medicine, University of Toronto; 2000:22–24.

V. SPECIAL SCENARIOS

Abdominal X-Ray
1. Lan F, Olscamp G. Practical aspects of the abdominal plain film in adults. *U Toronto Med J* 1997;75(1):16–22.

2. Yu R, Lan F, Weiser W. *Practical Radiology: The Chest X-Ray*. 1st ed. Toronto: University of Toronto Press; 1997: 120–122.

Angry Patient
1. Sachs P. Deflecting harsh words when tempers flare. *Nursing* 1999;29(3):62–64.

2. Sachs PR. Sticks and stones. How to respond when a patient's relatives take out their frustrations on you. *Nurse Manager* 1999;30(6):73–75.

Bad News
1. Balie W, Buckman R. *The Pocket Guide to Communication Skills in Clinical Practice, Including Breaking Bad News*. 1st ed. Toronto: Medical Audio Visual Communications; 1999.

Chest X-Ray
1. Lan F, Olscamp G. Practical aspects of the abdominal plain film in adults. *U Toronto Med J* 1997;75(1):16–22.

2. Yu R, Lan F, Weiser W. *Practical Radiology: The Chest X-Ray*. 1st ed. Toronto: University of Toronto Press; 1997: 3–36.

Chronic Disease
1. Rouse T, Tang G, Torgerson C, Van Spall H. *Essentials of Clinical Examination Handbook*. 3rd ed. Toronto: Medical Society Faculty of Medicine, University of Toronto; 2000:29–30.

Competency (Medical Decision Making)
1. Herbert, PC. *Doing Right: A Practical Guide to Ethics for Medical Trainees and Physicians*. 1st ed. New York: Oxford University Press; 1996: 153–173.

Elder Abuse
1. Wahl JA, Purdy S. *Elder Abuse: The Hidden Crime*. Toronto: Advocacy Centre for the Elderly; 1991:1–10.

Part VIII

Appendices

A. NORMAL LABRATORY VALUES

Table 1: Blood Chemistry*

Analyte	MGH Units	SI Units	Factor Conversion to SI
Ammonia	12–48 umol/L	12–48 umol/L	1.0
Bicarbonate	22–26 mEq/L	22–26 mEq/L	1.0
Bilirubin, direct	0.0–0.4 mg/dL	0–7 umol/L	17.1
Bilirubin, total	0.0–1.0 mg/dL	0–17 umol/L	17.1
Calcium	8.5–10.5 mg/dL	2.1–2.6 mmol/L	0.25
Calcium (ionized)	1.14–1.30 mmol/L	1.14–1.30 mmol/L	1.0
Chloride	100–108 mmol/L	100–108 mmol/L	1.0
Creatinine	0.6–1.5 mg/dL	53–133 umol/L	88.4
Glucose, Fasting	70–110 mg/dL	3.9–6.1 mmol/L	0.05551
HgB A1C	3.8–6.4%	0.038–0.064	0.01
Lactate	0.5–2.2 mmol/L	0.5–2.2 mmol/L	1.0
Magnesium	1.4–2.0 mEq/L	0.7–1.0 mmol/L	0.5
Osmolality	280–296 mOsm/kg	280–296 mOsm/kg	1.0
Phosphorous (inorganic)	2.6–4.5mg/dL	0.84–1.45 mmol/L	0.3229
Potassium	3.4–4.8 mmol/L	3.4–4.8 mmol/L	1.0
Urea Nitrogen	8–25 mg/dL	2.9–8.9 mmol/L	0.357
Uric Acid (male)	3.6–8.5 mg/dL	214–506 mol/L	59.48
Uric Acid (female)	2.3–6.6 mg/dL	137–393 mol/L	59.48

Table 2: Blood Enzymes, Hormones & Proteins*

Analyte	MGH Units	SI Units	Factor Conversion to SI
Alanine Aminotransferase (ALT, SGPT) -Male	10–55 U/L	0.17–0.92 ukat/L	
Alanine Aminotransferase (ALT, SGPT) -Female	7–30 U/L	0.12–0.50 ukat/L	
Albumin	3.1–4.3 g/dL	31–43 g/L	10.0
Adolase	0–7 U/L	0–7 U/L	1.0
Alkaline Phosphatase (ALP) -Male	45–115 U/L	0.75–1.92 ukat/L	0.01667
Alkaline Phosphatase (ALP) -Female	30–100 U/L	0.5–1.67 ukat/L	0.01667
Alpha-fetoprotein	<12.8 IU/mL	<9.92 ug/L	0.775
Amylase	53–123 U/L	0.88–2.05 nkat/L	0.01667
Aspartate Aminotransferase (AST) -Male	10–40 U/L	0.17–0.67 ukat/L	0.01667
Asparate Aminotransferase (AST) -Female	9–25 U/L	0.15–0.42 ukat/L	0.01667
Calcitonin -Male	3–26 pg/mL	3–26 ng/L	1.0
Calcitonin -Female	2–17 pg/mL	2–17 ng/L	1.0
Ceruloplasmin	27–50mg/dL	270–500 mg/L	10
Creatine Kinase -male	60–400 U/L	1.00–6.67 ukat/L	0.01667
Creatine Kinase -female	40–150 U/L	0.67–2.50 ukat/L	0.01667
Creatine Kinase, MB fraction	0–5 ug/mL	0–5 ug/mL	1.0
Globulin	2.6–4.1 g/dL	26–41 g/L	10
Glucagon	20–100 pg/mL	20–100 ng/L	1.0
Gamma-Glutamyltransferase -male	1–94 U/L	1–94 U/L	1.0
Gamma-Glutamyltransferase -female	1–70 U/L	1–70 U/L	1.0
Human Chorionic Gonadotropin (nonpregnant)	<5.0 mIU/mL	<5 IU/L	1.0
Lactate Dehydrogenase (LDH)	110–210 U/L	1.83–3.50 kat/L	0.01667
Lipase	3–19 U/dL	0.5–3.17 kat/L	0.1667
Prostate Specific Antigen (PSA) <40 y male	0.0–2.0 ng/mL	0.0–2.0 g/L	1.0
Prostate Specific Antigen (PSA) >40 y male	0.0–4.0 ng/mL	0.0–4.0 g/L	1.0
Protein, Total	6.0–8.0 g/dL	60–80 g/dL	10
Troponin I	<0.6 ng/mL	<0.6 g/L	1.0
Thyroid Stimulating Hormone	0.5–5.0 U/mL	0.5–5.0 U/mL	1.0
Thyroxine (T4)	4.5–10.9 g/dL	58–140 nmol/L	12.87
Triiodothyronine (T3)	60–181 ng/dL	0.92–2.78 nmol/L	0.01536

Table 3: Complete Blood Count, Differential & Coagulation Parameters*

Analyte	MGH Units	SI Units	Factor Conversion to SI
Bleed Time	2–9.5 min	2–9.5 min	1.0
D-Dimer	<0.5 g/mL	<0.5 g/mL	1.0
Differential Blood Count Neutrophils	45–75%	0.45–0.75	0.01
Differential Blood Count Bands	0–5%	0.0–0.05	0.01
Differential Blood Count Lymphocytes	16–46%	0.16–0.46	0.01
Differential Blood Count Monocytes	4–11%	0.04–0.11	0.01
Differential Blood Count Eosinophils	0–8%	0.0–0.8	0.01
Differential Blood Count Basophils	0–3%	0.0–0.03	0.01
Erthrocyte Count -male	4.50–5.30 X 10^6/mm3	4.50–5.30 X 10^{12}/L	1X106
Erthrocyte Count -female	4.10–5.10X 10^6/mm^3	4.10–5.10 X 10^{12}/L	1X106
Erthrocyte Sedimentation Rate (ESR) -Male	1–25 mm/h	1–25 mm/h	1.0
Erthrocyte Sedimentation Rate (ESR) -Male	1–17 mm/h	1–17 mm/h	1.0
Ferritin –male	30–300 ng/mL	30–300 g/L	1.0
Ferritin –female	10–200 ng/mL	10–200 g/L	1.0
Fibrinogen Degradation Products	<2.5 g/mL	<2.5mg/L	1.0
Fibrinogen	175–400 mg/dL	1.75–4.00 mol/L	0.01
Folate	3.1–17.5 ng/mL	7.0–39.7 nmol/L	2.266
Hemacrit -male	37.0–49.0	0.37–0.49	0.01
Hemacrit -female	36.0–46.0	0.36–0.46	0.01
Hemoglobin -male	13.0–18.0 g/dL	8.1–11.2 mmol/L	0.6206
Hemaglobin -female	12.0–16.0 g/dL	7.4–9.9 mmol/L	0.6206
Leukocytes (WBC)	4.5–11.0 X10^3/mm^3	4.5–11.0X10^9/L	1X10^6
Mean Corpuscular Hemoglobin (MCH)	25.0–35.0 pg/cell	25.0–35.0 pg/cell	1.0
Mean Corpscular Hemoglobin Concentration (MCHC)	31.0–37.0 g/dL	310–370 g/L	10
Mean Corpuscular Volume (MCV) -male	78–100 m^3	78–100 fL	1.0
Mean Corpuscular Volume (MCV) -female	78–102 m^3	78–102 fL	1.0
Partial-thromboplastin time, activated	22.1–34.1 s	22.1–34.1 s	1.0
Platelets	150–350X10^3/mm^3	150–350X10^6/L	1.0X10^6
Prothrombin time	11.2–13.2 s	11.2–13.2 s	1.0
Red-cell Distribution	11.5–14.5%	0.115–0.145	0.01
Reticulocyte	0.5–2.5% red cells	0.005–0.025 redcells	0.01
Thrombin Time	16–24 s	16–24 s	1.0
Vitamin B12	>250 pg/mL	>184 pmol/L	0.7378

*Values from above charts referenced from: Alexander Kratz, Kent B. Lewandrowski. 1998. MGH Case Records: Normal Reference Laboratory Values. NEJM 339(15),1063-10752

B. DERMATOME MAP

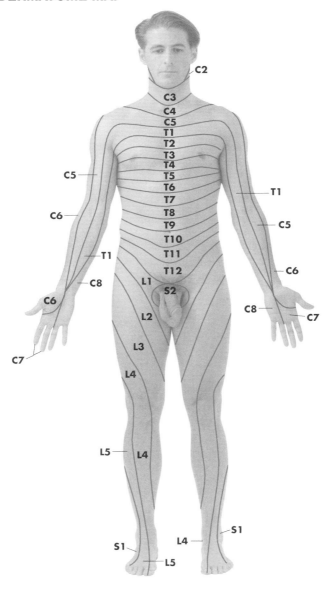

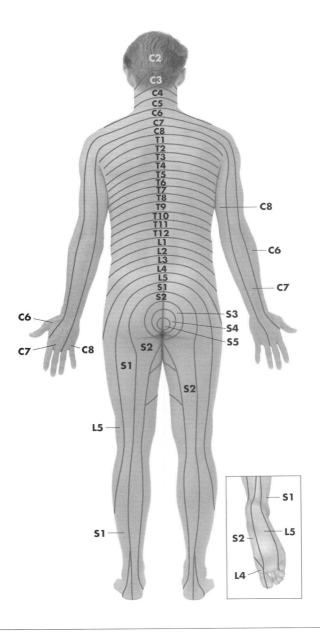

C. X-RAYS

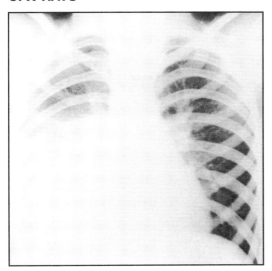

(A) Pneumonic consolidation of the right lower lobe. Posteroanterior view.

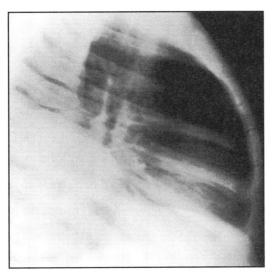

(B) Pneumonic consolidation of the right lower lobe. Lateral film.

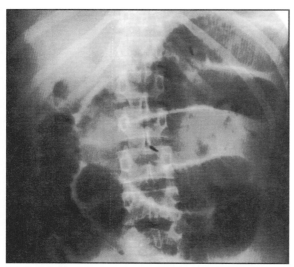

(C) Small bowel obstruction: supine film showing dilated loops of small bowel in step-ladder pattern

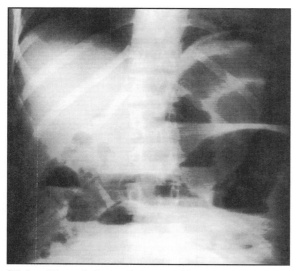

(D) Small bowel obstruction: erect film showing air fluid levels

Appendix C Source: Sutton, D., *Radiology and Imaging for Medical Students*, 7th ed. (London: Churchill Livingstone), pp. 29, 30, and 143.

D. Brand Names in Canada, Australia, and the United States

Generic Name	Brand Name		
	Canada	Australia	United States
acarbose	Prandase	Glucobay	Precose
acetaminophen	Atasol Tempra	Panadol Paracetamol Tylenol	Atasol Tempra Tylenol
acetylcysteine	Mucomyst	Mucomyst	Mucomyst
allopurinol	Zyloprim	Zyloprim (several others)	Aloprim Zyloprim
amantadine HCl	Endantadine	Symmetrel Gen-Amantadine Symmetrel	Symadine Symmetrel
amikacin	Amikin	Amikin	Amikin
amphotericin B	Fungizone	Ambisome Fungilin Oral Fungizone	Amphocin Fungizone
ampicillin	Ampicin Penbritin	Alphacin Ampicyn Austrapen	Ampicin Penbritin
anileridine	Leritine	NA	NA
ASA (acetylsalicylic acid)	Aspirin Entrophen (several others)	Aspro Disprin Spren (several others)	Aspirin Entrophen (several others)
atorvastatin calcium	Lipitor	Lipitor	Lipitor
atropine sulphate	Isopto Atropine Minims Atropine	Minims	Atro-Pen
azithromycin	Zithromax	Zithromax	Zithromax
baclofen	(several others) Lioresal	Lioresal	Lioresal
Benzhexol hydrochloride	Apo-Trihex Trihexiphenidyl Hydrochloride	Artane	Artane Trihexane
bromocriptine mesylate	Parlodel	Bromolactin Kripton Parlodel	Parlodel
captopril	Capoten	Capoten	Capoten
carbenicillin disodium	Pyopen	NA	Geopen
carbidopa/ levodopa	Sinemet	Sinemet	Sinemet
cefaclor	Apo-Cefaclor Ceclor	Ceclor	Ceclor
cefazolin sodium (cephazolin [Aus])	Ancef Kefzol	Kefzol	Ancef Kefzol
cefotetan disodium	Cefotan	Apatef	Cefotan
ceftizoxime sodium	Cefizox	NA	Cefizox
ceftriaxone sodium	Rocephin	Rocephin	Rocephin

continued

Generic Name	Brand Name		
	Canada	Australia	United States
cefuroxime axetil (oral)	Ceftin	Zinnat	Ceftin
cefuroxime sodium (injectable)	Kefurox Zinacef	NA	Kefurox Zinacef
cephalexin	Keflex	Keflex	Keflex
cephalothin	Ceporacin	Keflin	NA
chlorpromazine HCl	Largactil	Largactil	Thorazine
clarithromycin	Biaxin	Klacid	Biaxin
clomiphene citrate	Clomid Serophene	Clomexal Clomid Serophene	Clomid Milophene Serophene
clopidogrel hydrogen sulfate	Plavix Plavix	Iscover	Plavix
estrogens (conjugated)	Premarin	Premarin	Congest Premarin
cyanocobalamin (injectable)	Cobalamin	Cytamen	several
cyclophosphamide	Cytoxan Procytox	Cycloblastin Endoxan	Cytoxan Neosar
dalteparin sodium	Fragmin	Fragmin	Fragmin
danazol	Cyclomen	Azol Danocrine	Danocrine
dexamethasone (oral)	Decadron Deronil Dexasone Maxidex Oradexon	Decadron (injection) Dexmethsone Maxidex	Decadron Dexone Hexadrol
diclofenac sodium	Voltaren	Voltaren	Voltaren
digoxin	Lanoxin	Lanoxin Sigmaxin	Lanoxicaps Lanoxin
digoxin immune Fab	Digibind	Digibind	Digibind Digidote
dihydroergotamine mesylate	Migranal	Dihydergot	D.H.E. 45
diltiazem	Cardizem	Auscard Cardizem	Cardizem
dimenhydrinate	Gravol Dramamine	Dramamine	Dimetabs Dramamine Gravol
diphenhydramine HCl	Benadryl	Benadryl	Benadryl
docusate sodium	Colace Soflax	Coloxyl	Colace Regulax
donepezil HCl	Aricept	Aricept	Aricept
dopamine	Intropin	dopamine	Intropin
epinephrine HCl	Adrenalin Vaponefrin	Adrenaline	Adrenalin

continued

Generic Name	Brand Name		
	Canada	Australia	United States
erythromycin (several forms)	(several others) Erythromid	Erythrocin	(several others) E-Mycin
fentanyl citrate	fentanyl citrate	Sublimaze	Sublimaze
fentanyl (transdermal patch)	Duragesic	Duragesic	Duragesic
fluconazole	Diflucan	Diflucan	Diflucan
flumazenil	Anexate	Anexate	Romazicon
5-fluorouracil	Adrucil Efudex Fluorouracil	Efudix	Adrucil Efudex
fluphenazine decanoate	Modecate	Anatensol Modecate	
fluphenazine HCl			Prolixin
furosemide (frusemide)	Lasix	Lasix Urex	Lasix
gentamicin	Cidomycin Garamycin	Gentamicin	Garamycin
gliclazide	Diamicron	Diamicron Glyade Nidem	NA
glyburide	Diaßeta (several others)	NA	Diaßeta
heparin sodium	Hepalean Heparin Leo	heparin injection	heparin injection
hydrochlorothiazide	HydroDiuril	Dichlotride	HydroDiuril
hydrocortisone	Cortef	Hysone	Cortef
hydrocortisone sodium succinate	Solu-Cortef	Solu-Cortef	Solu-Cortef
hydroxyzine	Atarax	NA	Hyzine Vistaril
ibuprofen	Advil Motrin	Brufen Nurofen Rafen	Advil Motrin
indinavir sulfate	Crixivan	Crixivan	
indomethacin	Indocid	Indocid	Indocin
ipratropium bromide	Apo-Ipravent Atrovent Novo-Ipramide	Atrovent	Atrovent
isoproterenol HCl	Isuprel	isoprenaline Isuprel	Isuprel
ketorolac tromethamine	Acular Toradol	Acular Toradol	Acular Toradol
levonorgestrel	Mirena Plan B	Microlut Microval Mirena Postinor-2	Norplant

continued

Generic Name	Brand Name		
	Canada	Australia	United States
levothyroxine sodium	Eltroxin Synthroid	Oroxine	Eltroxin Synthroid
lidocaine HCl (lignocaine)	Lidodan Xylocaine	Xylocaine	Dilocaine Xylocaine (several others)
lisinopril	Prinivil Zestril	Prinivil Zestril	Prinivil Zestril
lorazepam	Ativan	Ativan	Ativan
maprotiline	Ludiomil	NA	Ludiomil
mefenamic acid	Ponstan	Mefic Ponstan	Ponstel
meperidine HCl (pethidine HCl)	Demerol	pethidine	Demerol
metformin HCl	Glucophage	Diamex Glucomet Glucophage (several others)	Glucophage
methylprednisolone	Medrol		Medrol
methylprednisolone acetate	Depo-Medrol	Depo-Medrol	Depo-Medrol
methylprednisolone sodium succinate	Solu-Medrol	Solu-Medrol	Solu-Medrol
metronidazole	Flagyl	Flagyl	Flagyl Metro IV
misoprostol	Cytotec	Cytotec	Cytotec
morphine sulfate	Kadian M-Eslon MS-Contin Statex	Anamorph Kapanol	Astramorph PF Duramorph Roxanol (several others)
nadolol	Corgard	NA	Corgard
naloxone HCl	Narcan	Narcan	Narcan
naproxen	Naprosyn	Inza Naprosyn Proxen	Naprosyn (several others)
naproxen sodium	NA	Anaprox Naprogesix	NA
nitroglycerin	(several others)	(several others)	(several others)
norethindrone acetate	Norlutate	NA	Micronor Nor-QD
nystatin	Mycostatin Nadostine Nilstat PMS-Nystatin	Mycostatin Nilstat	Mycostatin Nilstat Nystex
olanzapine	Zyprexa	Zyprexa	Zyprexa
orlistat	Xenical	Xenical	Xenical
pantoprazole	Pantoloc	Somac	Protonix

continued

Generic Name	Brand Name		
	Canada	Australia	United States
penicillin G potassium	NA	NA	Pfizerpen
penicillin G benzathine	Megacillin	Bicillin	Bicillin Bicillin Megacillin Wycillin
penicillin G procaine	Ayercillin		
penicillin V potassium	(several others) Ledercillin VK	(several others)	Pen-Vee K Ledercillin VK V-Cillin K
pericyazine	Neuleptil	Neulactil	NA
perphenazine	Trilafon	NA	Trilafon
phenobarbital	generic	phenobarbitone	Generic
phenytoin	Dilantin	Dilantin	Dilantin
pneumococcal 7-valent conjugate vaccine	Prevnar	Prevenar	Prevnar
potassium chloride	(several others) Slow-K Kay Ciel	(several others)	Kaon-CL (several others)
procainamide	Procan SR Pronestyl	Pronestyl	Procan SR Pronestyl
pyrazinamide	Tebrazid	Zinamide	PMS Pyrazinamide
pyrimethamine	Daraprim	Daraprim	Daraprim
quinapril	Accupril	Accupril	Accupril
repaglinide	GlucoNorm	NovoNorm	Prandin
rifabutin	Mycobutin	Mycobutin	Mycobutin
rifampin (rifampicin)	Rifadin Rofact	Rifadin Rimycin	Rifadin Rimactane
rosiglitazone maleate	Avandia	Avandia	Avandia
salbutamol (albuterol)	Ventolin	Ventolin	Ventolin
selegiline hydrochloride	Eldepryl	Eldepryl Selgene	Carbex Eldepryl SD-Deprenyl
sildenafil citrate	Viagra	Viagra	Viagra
spironolactone	Aldactone	Aldactone Spiractin	Aldactone
sulfasalazine	Alti-Sulfasalazine PMS-Sulfasalazine Salazopyrin	Salazopyrin	Azulfidine
sumatriptan succinate	Imitrex	Imigran Suvalan	Imitrex
tamoxifen citrate	Nolvadex Tamofen	Nolvadex Tamosin Tamoxen	Nalvodex
theophylline	Theo-Dur Theolair	Theo-Dur	Theo-Dur Theolair

continued

Generic Name	Brand Name		
	Canada	Australia	United States
tinzaparin sodium	Innohep	NA	Innohep
trazodone HCl	Desyrel	NA	Desyrel
warfarin sodium	Coumadin Marevan	Coumadin	Coumadin
zopiclone	Imovane	Imovane	NA

(NA = not available)